POLICY AND PRACTICE IN EDUCATION

NUMBER TWENTY-SEVEN

PHYSICAL EDUCATION: PICKING UP THE BATON

POLICY AND PRACTICE IN EDUCATION

1:   Lindsay Paterson, *Education and the Scottish Parliament* (out of print)

2:   Gordon Kirk, *Enhancing Quality in Teacher Education* (out of print)

3:   Nigel Grant, *Multicultural Education in Scotland* (out of print)

4:   Lyn Tett, *Community Education, Lifelong Learning and Social Inclusion* (Second edition, 2006)

5:   Sheila Riddell, *Special Educational Needs: Providing Additional Support* (Second edition, 2006)

6:   J. Eric Wilkinson, *Early Childhood Education: The New Agenda* (2003)

7:   Henry Maitles, *Values in Education: We're All Citizens Now* (2005)

8:   Willis Pickard and John Dobie, *The Political Context of Education after Devolution* (2003)

9:   Jim O'Brien, Daniel Murphy and Janet Draper, *School Leadership* (2003)

10:   Margaret Nicolson and Matthew MacIver (eds), *Gaelic Medium Education* (2003)

11:   Gordon Kirk, Walter Beveridge and Iain Smith, *The Chartered Teacher* (2003)

12:   Jim O'Brien and Gale Macleod, *The Social Agenda of the School* (2009)

13:   Ann Glaister and Bob Glaister (eds), *Inter-Agency Collaboration: Providing for Children* (2005)

14:   Mary Simpson, *Assessment* (2005)

15:   Ian Menter, Estelle Brisard and Ian Smith, *Convergence or Divergence? Initial Teacher Education in Scotland and England* (2006)

16:   Janet Draper and Jim O'Brien, *Induction: Fostering Career Development at All Stages* (2006)

17:   Sheila Riddell and Lyn Tett, *Gender and Teaching: Where Have All the Men Gone?* (2006)

18:   George Head, *Better Learning, Better Behaviour* (2007)

19:   Margaret Martin, *Building a Learning Community in the Primary Classroom* (2007)

20:   Christine Forde (ed.), *Tackling Gender Inequality, Raising Pupil Achievement* (2007)

21:   Daniel Murphy, *Professional School Leadership, Dealing with Dilemmas* (2007)

22:   Beth Dickson and James McGonigal, *Creativity, Culture and Community* (2008)

23:   Stephen J. McKinney (ed.), *Faith Schools in the Twenty-First Century* (2008)

24:   Jenny Reeves and Alison Fox (eds), *Practice-Based Learning: Developing Excellence in Teaching* (2008)

25:   Jeannie Mackenzie, *Family Learning, Engaging with Parents* (2009)

26:   Margery McMahon, *International Education: Educating for a Global Future* (2009)

27:   Malcolm Thorburn and Shirley Gray, *Physical Education: Picking up the Baton* (2009)

POLICY AND PRACTICE IN EDUCATION

SERIES EDITORS

JIM O'BRIEN and **CHRISTINE FORDE**

PHYSICAL EDUCATION: PICKING UP THE BATON

Malcolm Thorburn

*Lecturer, Moray House School of Education,
University of Edinburgh*

and

Shirley Gray

*Lecturer, Moray House School of Education,
University of Edinburgh*

DUNEDIN

Published by
Dunedin Academic Press Ltd
Hudson House
8 Albany Street
Edinburgh EH1 3QB
Scotland

ISBN: 978-1-906716-07-3
ISSN 1479-6910

British Library Cataloguing in Publication data
A catalogue record for this book is available from the British Library

Typeset by Makar Publishing Production
Printed in the United Kingdom by Cpod, Trowbridge, Wiltshire
Printed on paper from sustainable resources

Mixed Sources
Product group from well-managed
forests and other controlled sources
www.fsc.org Cert no. TT-COC-2082
© 1996 Forest Stewardship Council
FSC

CONTENTS

Series editors' introduction   *vi*

Chapter 1: Opportunities and challenges for physical education   1
Malcolm Thorburn

Chapter 2: Official and unofficial views of physical education   8
Malcom Thorburn

Chapter 3: Teaching physical education in the twenty-first
century: pedagogical challenges   30
Shirley Gray

Chapter 4: Professionalism and professional development   48
Malcom Thorburn and Shirley Gray

Chapter 5: What future for physical education?   68
Malcolm Thorburn

References   78

Index   88

SERIES EDITORS' INTRODUCTION

This volume in the Policy and Practice in Education series charts developments in the area of physical education. The subject has evolved in recent years to occupy a central place in secondary education and its importance is similarly evident in primary schools with the rapid expansion of specialist teaching in physical education. The thrust of policy in the areas of education, health and sport pose significant challenges. In their critique of these policy imperatives, Malcolm Thorburn and Shirley Gray illustrate how these tensions can impact on teachers involved in designing and teaching physical education programmes. Teachers are faced with competing demands; for example, the nurturing of elite sporting talent and at the same time the fostering of habits of active lifestyles in all. There is a danger that in the struggle to deal with these tensions the core concern on the quality of learning is lost. Here the authors establish the importance of meaningful learning experiences for pupils.

The authors provide a clear analysis of pedagogic practices and assessment processes in physical education, demonstrating that a concern for pupil-centred approaches not only enriches pupilsí experiences of the subject but brings with it benefits for wider achievement and personal well being. These high expectations of physical education demand much of teachers in terms of their skills and understanding. In the final sections of this book, the focus turns to the question of the role and development of physical education teachers. Here the authors draw from their experiences as teacher educators to provide a thought-provoking review of the implications of these changes for the preparation and continuing development of teachers working in the different school sectors.

Dr Jim O'Brien
Professor of Leadership & Professional Learning, Dean and Director, Moray House School of Education, The University of Edinburgh

Christine Forde
Professor of Leadership & Professional Learning, Department of Educational Studies, Faculty of Education, The University of Glasgow

CHAPTER 1

Opportunities and Challenges for Physical Education

Introduction

Physical education as a subject in the school curriculum has often presented something of a paradox; for while the subject has been included in curriculum for many years, the reasons why has often not been entirely clear (Kirk, 1988). Yet, despite being a familiar and well established subject, views about the aims and benefits of physical education are often polarised and highly contested. Politicians, the media, parents and pupils, as well as teachers and student teachers of physical education, have varied and contrasting views about the subject. So, in the future quite how physical education will be experienced by pupils and how the professional needs and requirements of teachers will be met are important considerations to review, if physical education is to be successful in capitalising on many of the policy opportunities which currently exist.

Accordingly, the main aim of the book is to help readers comprehend, in greater detail, some of the reasons why physical education is so contested and generally a more complex concern than might be initially anticipated. To provide a framework for analysis and review, the three central themes of the book are discussed in three specific main chapters.

❑ Chapter 2 focuses on how policy in physical education has been explained in official policy documents as well as reviewing 'unofficial' accounts of how effective policy reporting has been in advancing coherent arguments for physical education programmes.

❑ Chapter 3 focuses on the teaching of physical education and the changes which should be considered if the pedagogical approaches teachers adopt are to support curriculum in physical education in future years.

❑ Chapter 4 focuses on professionalism and professional development within physical education and addresses concerns about how the professional needs of teachers can best be met in future years.

The policy – pedagogy – professionalism priorities most influencing physical education at this time is contextualised through discussing these challenges in conjunction with the precise aims and intentions of different curriculum programmes.

The central themes of the book

Policy in physical education

The process of creating policy is often shaped and influenced by degrees of conflict and compromise with some eventual form of negotiated or partially agreed resolution eventually informing official policy announcements (Ball, 2008). Furthermore, stakeholders in the policy process are rarely equal. Those formally invited to be involved, for example, representatives from public bodies such as Learning and Teaching Scotland (LTS), the Scottish Qualifications Authority (SQA) and Her Majesty's Inspectorate of Education (HMIE) plus invited teachers, tend to occupy a rather privileged position under the largely patronage-based model of policy development favoured in Scotland (Humes, 2008). Therefore, other interested voices can remain outside of the formal policy making apparatus; for example, academics, teachers, parents and pupils, and representatives from smaller organisations are not usually invited to join formal policy making groups, even though these individuals and groups have various perspectives on the best way forward for physical education. Unsurprisingly, in this environment, the ways in which policy impacts on practice is rarely as smooth or straightforward as anticipated.

Accordingly, in a text of this sort, it is important that 'unofficial' voices are reviewed in order that the policy language and 'narrative privilege' of official policy reporting is not assumed or presented as being the only position it is possible to adopt (Humes, 2008, p. 71). This position is particularly required within the context of a single subject – physical education – for at this level provided the formal outcomes of the policy process articulate with the curriculum prerequisites of the day, in terms of adopting the common language of 'outcomes', 'capacities' or whatever, then official policy has the potential to operate in relatively autonomous ways when making important decisions about the aims, values and future directions of a subject. Consequently, it is worth critiquing the areas of policy which are most contested and the policy solutions which are proposed for addressing the challenges identified. A further issue for physical education, which adds to the complexity of matters at this time, is that the single-subject status of physical education might be set for a degree of change due to recent policy intentions to cluster similar subjects together in the school curriculum. In addition, the ways in which school agendas dovetail with the communities' schools serve are likely to come under review in the future and this might impact as well on the practice of physical education.

Overall, policy can be conceived of as operating within a crowded space (Houlihan and Green, 2006), where different interest groups within education, health and sport seek to promote their particular values and aspirations. So, as will become apparent in discussions in Chapter 2, physical education has to co-exist alongside policy goals aimed at improving school ethos, academic attainment, health improvement as well as the development of participation and excellence in sport. Inevitably this makes finding a coherent policy approach for delivering on all of these goals difficult for the various groups devising related education, health and sport policies, as some goals are not necessarily entirely compatible or consistent with each other. One consequence of this difficulty is that policy communities search for evidence to justify policy and practice, even though this frequently remains difficult to find. Coalter (2007) for example, highlights that due to various conceptual, methodological and situational weaknesses, there is often a lack of adequate research informing policy and practice. A second policy difficulty is that policy implementation can show signs of slippage, as what is intended to occur is somewhat different from that which actually ends up happening in practice. Therefore, in summary, given the raft of policy changes which might be afoot in future years, Chapter 2 aims to analyse the adequacy of the goals set for physical education with discussion focusing on the consequences policy might have on the practice of physical education.

Pedagogy in physical education

Recent policy developments within education and physical education present many challenges for teachers in terms of interpreting policy documentation and organising and delivering new curriculum. These difficulties are likely to be particularly acute if policy aims are counter to teachers' experiences and beliefs about curriculum and teaching. Additionally, when there is a lack direction, or when support documentation does not provide teachers with sufficient detail about the application of policy, very little change is likely to occur in the ways teachers deliver the curriculum.

The new challenges in teaching are particularly focused on encouraging a greater sense of responsibility, autonomy and independence in pupils and in helping pupils to improve their self-confidence when working collaboratively (HMIE, 2008). These attributes can best be developed if teachers adopt more pupil-centred teaching approaches, making content more meaningful, with pupils developing their ability to think critically, solve problems and transfer their learning to a variety of contexts. In these learning environments, pupils become more interested and more engaged.

From this perspective, learning in physical education is supported by more complex theories of learning, for example, constructivism (Oslin and Mitchell, 2006) and situated learning (Kirk and MacPhail, 2002), both of which emphasise the interactions of the learner within the environment in the construction of knowledge. The broader range of outcomes that constructivist teaching appears to afford, and the potential links it has to curriculum aims, are evidenced through teaching approaches such as Sport Education (Siedentop, 1994), Teaching Games for Understanding (TGfU) (Bunker and Thorpe, 1982) and the Tactical approach (Griffin *et al.*, 1997). These are pupil-centred teaching approaches that focus on the context for learning, thus providing pupils with more authentic and meaningful experiences. With such teaching approaches, the teacher has a less direct role in the learning process, employing strategies such as question and answer, modified game and problem-solving tasks, thus giving pupils more responsibility for their own learning.

However, disappointingly a great deal of teaching in physical education has been predominantly teacher-led (Capel, 2007), where there is a focus on providing pupils with information which facilitates the development of technically proficient performances of specific skills. Teachers teach in this way because they believe that pupils cannot successfully access physical activities unless they are able to perform the techniques of that activity first. However, although pupils can become technically proficient within this learning context, when they have to apply skills in a more authentic context, they are presented with new and more difficult problems to solve. This can result in a poor transfer of skills and overall have a negative impact on pupils' motivation to learn. Moreover, because the practice environment is so different from the performance environment, pupils do not see the purpose, or the relevance, of the skills they are completing. These factors are detrimental to the progress pupils can make in physical education and is of concern as research suggests that those pupils who are less skilful are more likely to drop out of physical activity and lead sedentary lifestyles during adulthood (Standage *et al.*, 2007).

Therefore, the main purpose of Chapter 3 is to highlight the challenges involved in pursuing pedagogical change. In attempting to fulfil this remit, Chapter 3 explores the role of teachers' beliefs about teaching, as well as their knowledge of the theories that support teaching and learning. This is important as a starting point, because if change is to take place, then teachers need to be more critical of their current practices and develop their knowledge and understanding of alternative, pupil-centred approaches to teaching, approaches which are framed by constructivist theories of teaching and learning.

Professionalism in physical education

Chapter 4 focuses on the main professionalism challenges ahead in physical education and the types of opportunities and experiences which it might be useful to include within teacher education programmes and professional development programmes for experienced teachers. These challenges are pertinent to explore, given the new centrality of physical education and the policy expectation that programmes in schools can articulate with the requirements of society to increase lifetime physical activity and learning, and also contribute towards achieving greater standards of sporting excellence.

However, as will be discussed in this chapter, there are often difficulties in mapping out how best to transfer policy intentions into worthwhile professional development programmes. The vexed issue of the extent of student teachers experiences of practical activities (Hepburn, 2009) is one particularly animated concern; a concern which tends to be exacerbated further by the general sense that the academic world of theory is considered as rather dislocated from the professional world of teaching. Furthermore, professionally related programmes have often had to grapple with the complexities of advising teachers to continue to be reflective about their contribution to learning and to whole school improvement, while at the same time recognising that professional development programmes need to meet the latest accountability requirements of national government and local authorities. Thus, improving professionalism takes place against a challenging policy backdrop and against increasing use of identified targets for greater learning gains to be achieved across the different ages and stages of schooling. Consequently, fundamental issues exist about how professional programmes at initial teacher level and for experienced teachers can best be conceived and delivered. Therefore, a main focus of this chapter is on analysing the conceptual and implementation issues most associated with providing support for these key stages of professionalism.

In addition, just as physical education teachers have to recognise the range of contrasting curriculum objectives which exist, it is also important that teachers are alert to the changing expectations of the health and sporting communities in developing effective working partnerships with the profession. For this reason quite how physical education teachers might in years to come share responsibilities across a range of school and community wide initiatives are reviewed. This is especially important to review at this time, as teachers are adapting to new conditions of service agreements. Additionally, the reasons influencing pupils' participation interests are becoming an ever more complex factor to consider when reviewing the practice of physical education in school and youth sport during out of school hours.

Following these three main chapters, the concluding chapter (Chapter 5) draws together some of the main policy – pedagogy – professionalism themes and issues most influencing physical education at this time.

The structure of the book

The main purpose of the text is explanatory and analytical. While critical questions are raised, overt personal opinions and value judgements are as far as reasonably possible not included in the text. What it intended, by contrast, is that some of the assumptions upon which policy, pedagogy and professionalism have been developed are reviewed, so that the changing influences on physical education in terms policy, pedagogy and professionalism, and in terms of the curriculum aims which have been ascribed to various programmes can be understood with greater clarity.

Decisions have also been taken about a suitable starting point for the book. For the most part, analysis focuses on the period from the 1970s onwards until the present day. Since this time many common policies and practices have operated until the present day. Noteworthy among these is recognition that:

- The majority of state secondary schools are run on comprehensive rather than selection-based principles.
- The school leaving age has remained at 16.
- The curriculum and assessment reviews within secondary schools (Munn and Dunning reports) which created Standard Grades courses are still mostly in operation.
- Graduate degree programmes are still used as the main requirement for entry into the teaching profession.

While these factors influenced the timescale selected, trying to secure an equally precise definition of physical education would have proved much more problematic. As such, in order to accommodate related viewpoints and to ensure that physical education arguments are suitably contextualised, the book includes, where appropriate related agendas and issues pertaining to health and well-being and youth sport. This approach is necessary because it appears highly likely that debates in these areas of policy will influence the increasingly politicised world of physical education in years to come. For these reasons, it is necessary that reviews of physical education take account of how new devolutionary powers have been used to improve the centrality of health and well-being within schools and the role that physical education might be expected to occupy within such a remit. Equally, the capacity of success in sport to nourish nationalistic pride cannot be overlooked and therefore the impact of agendas for developing sporting talent without compromising educational principles merits review in a text of this sort as well.

Two other points of clarity are worthwhile to explain at this point. Firstly, we have tried as far as possible to refer to 'pupils' when discussing primary and secondary age schooling. When discussing out of school learning in health and sporting communities we have predominantly used the term 'young people'. Secondly, various stakeholders in the policy process have undergone changes of title over the years. We have used the title which was in existence at the time of policy announcements. So, for example, we refer to the Scottish Executive for the period between 1999 and 2007 and the Scottish Government from 2008 onwards.

CHAPTER 2

Official and Unofficial Views of Physical Education

Synopsis

The aim of this chapter is to analyse the contested arguments which have surrounded debates about the nature and purposes of physical education in the last thirty years in Scotland. Various points of contention are discussed in the light of official policy documents and unofficial reporting on physical education by teachers, academics and politicians informing review. The intention is that the chapter will provide a critical introduction which contextualises the curriculum, pedagogical and professional development challenges discussed in later chapters.

Introduction

During the early 1970s physical education existed in a 'world of its own' where the predominant focus of teachers' reflections was on subject-specific issues (Thomson, 1993, p. 6). However, by the mid 1970s, physical education like other subjects was required to review its aims and intentions in light of the changing political, social and economic circumstances which began to impact on education policy and schooling (Anderson, 1999). The educational endorsement of physical activity in the Munn Report was well received by physical educationalists, given the unease which has often existed among the profession about the marginal role of the subject (Brewer and Sharp, 1999). Yet, rather than lead as expected to the increased profile of 'core' physical education programmes for pupils in the middle years of secondary schooling, the later implementation of policy led to the introduction of examination awards at Standard Grade level. Therefore, by the late 1980s dual forms of provision existed: for most pupils, physical education consisted of little over an hour each week of core physical education and, in addition, pupils could choose to complete an examination award in the subject as well.

The development of various examination awards tended to dominate policy space during the late 1980s and 1990s; their introduction opening up a range of new curriculum opportunities as well as highlighting a number of pedagogical and professional development concerns. During this period, core physical education programmes tended to become adversely affected by a lack of time and curriculum prominence. However, the fortunes of the subject changed markedly at the turn of the century, as evidence of declining health across the school age population triggered the need for interventions to address identified problems. Physical education as part of health and well-being became pivotal to delivering the aims of a 'Curriculum for Excellence' (CfE). Away from the immediacies of the school day, various policy initiatives have identified physical activity and youth sport as a beneficial part of out of hours schooling.

Taking all of the above into account, the chapter will focus predominantly on:

- the introduction and development of examination awards in physical education;
- the changing fortunes of core physical education programmes;
- physical education, health and well-being and a curriculum for excellence;
- physical activity and youth sport

The introduction and development of examination awards in physical education

The rationale within examination awards at Standard Grade and Higher level has been to integrate 'performance' with 'knowledge and understanding' or 'analysis of performance'. The intention is that through rich practice-based experiential learning, pupils can improve standards of practical performance and their understanding of associated content knowledge and analysis processes which underpin performance improvement. The commitment towards an integrated learning approach is reflected in the assessment arrangements, where there is an equal (or near equal) weighting between practical performance and analytical understanding as measured by written assessment answers. Consequently, what is intended is that productive learning environments with time for note making, completion of task sheets, data collection and so on will dovetail with learning about how to improve performance. For teachers, achieving a connectivity where 'practice reveals knowledge' and 'knowledge informs practice' is necessary for authentic learning: authentic in the sense that learning is in keeping with the spirit of the rationale for examination awards.

In pursuing these aims policy makers were, in effect, arguing that with some careful adjustment physical education could be accommodated within an academic conception of education. Crucial to success is keeping the spirit of practical experiential learning alive while also achieving high levels of attainment in formal national examinations. As Bilsborough and MacLeod (1998, p. 23) note:

> Teachers took it for granted that physical activity would be the nucleus of any Standard Grade Course. There was never any possibility that they would entertain a classroom based, academic study of physical education – a route which some colleagues in England had followed.

During the development of examination awards the influence of lecturers at teacher training institutions was modest relative to the role of HMIE whose directives in shaping policy became more important (Thomson, 1993). Under the auspices of HMIE, seconded teachers as development officers worked to produce support materials and lead professional development programmes. This was a challenging remit, especially when the multiple levels of the Higher Still framework of awards were devised during the mid 1990s. Humes (1999) considers that using seconded teachers can be an untidy and frustrating model for implementing policy as development officers have to satisfy two divergent audiences – those of the policy community at national level, and, practising teachers at a local level. Unsurprisingly, MacPhail (2007) found, specifically within higher level physical education, that the lack of understanding between policy makers and teachers created tensions about expected levels of support and assistance as implementation continued: a commentary endorsed by numerous teacher contributions to the *Scottish Journal of Physical Education*, for example, Douglas (1998, p. 49) urged policy makers to provide relevant in-service training about the underpinning content knowledge associated with integrated teaching and learning so that 'we ourselves can answer the questions that are set!'

The extent of the implementation concerns became exacerbated further as adverse comment began to emerge about the quality of the teaching approaches adopted, with HMIE reporting that:

> Too many teachers resort to the classroom, a 'talk and chalk' approach and the use of simple worksheets. This is in contrast to the spirit of ... a practical-experiential approach to the development of knowledge and understanding ... [which] ... should be developed in practical contexts, ideally with pupils working on different levels of practical tasks which allow them to display and develop their practical understanding. (SOED/HMIE, 1995, 5.29)

Brewer and Sharp (1999, p. 544) refer to the terseness of this statement as 'comment approaching rebuke', even though the statement is contained within an overall report others consider to be 'deliberately non-judgemental' (Thomson, 1996, p. 42), and which 'painted a relatively uncritical picture of the status quo' (Bilsborough and MacLeod, 1998, p. 25). Overall, evidence was beginning to emerge of a gap between policy expectations as monitored by the HMIE, and the ability of teachers to deliver the standards of attainment expected through practical experiential teaching and learning approaches. Due to the emergence of these operational difficulties in deploying the rationale, the development of content knowledge and the imbalance in levels of attainment between performance and analytical abilities are particularly worthy of more detailed review.

The development of content knowledge

Due to the broad range of definitions of physical education which exist it was always likely that the introduction of examination awards would invoke some degree of contestation. At its simplest, it is often difficult to gain agreement on a definition of physical education when the subject area has natural and feasible points of connection with the 'arts', the 'sciences' and with 'personal and social education'. Furthermore, the favouring of one area over another creates the impression of distortion and a reduction of the pluralist values which could feasibly be ascribed to physical education (Reid, 1997). Kirk (2002) notes that it was perceptual-motor skills and games statements rather than aesthetic references to performance, which informed the introduction of examination awards at Standard Grade level; a position which if nothing else matched most teachers preferred values at this time (Sharp, 1990).

During the Higher Still programme this area was revisited and teachers were invited to introduce a more rounded view of performance (performance appreciation) as the starting point for a more personalised and detailed analysis of performance. However, this was rarely selected by teachers as a beneficial addition to their courses with assessment answers at national level remaining few in number and quality. MacPhail (2007, p. 52) found when summarising teachers' views about whether to introduce higher level awards or not that 'no teacher voiced support for the flexibility' available in the supporting arrangements document. Thus, in this complex policy setting, development officers had the difficult task of trying to clarify and nudge forwards developments in content knowledge which reflected the emerging nature and diverse potential of the subject area, while also attempting to recognise teachers' apparent desire for greater support and course prescription.

The nature of the content knowledge defined in arrangements documents and the degree of teacher choice available within courses raises a number of associated points and uppermost among these is how will the multiple voices of pupils be recognised? This is a particular concern with regard to the quality of girls learning experiences in examination awards; for while nearly a third of pupils select Standard Grade physical education the gender balance has changed little over the last two decades with generally 70% of those completing awards being male. And, while scrutiny of assessment results indicates very little difference in levels of attainment realised, in some quarters the gendered nature of content knowledge and the way in which schools have constructed their courses has invoked criticism (Menzies, 1997; 1998). Additionally, Further Education lecturers have often been uneasy about the narrowness of examination award provision due to the limited focus on performance improvement. It has been argued that offering a range of different awards would better link physical education in schools with more vocationally inclined awards in health and exercise and sports coaching and development. In this respect, it could be that the Higher Still programme of reform was not radical enough with the awards designed in physical education being rather one-dimensional (Thorburn, 2004).

The imbalance in attainment between performance and analytical abilities

A major problem with examination awards is that pupils have always performed markedly better in practical rather than analytical areas. For many years at higher level the differences were particularly acute with pupils' regularly gaining over four-fifths of the marks available for performance but little over two-fifths of the marks available in analytical areas. Clearly, the majority of pupils can achieve a high practical performance standard, although when asked to articulate their thoughts through written answers, their work is often poor or modest.

MacPhail (2007) found that only a third of teachers (32%) considered that the pedagogical approaches recommended were realistic with nearly two-thirds (59%) of teachers who were not planning to introduce higher level awards citing lack of staff development as the most significant factor influencing their decision. Brewer and Sharp (1999, p. 543) indicate that the degree to which the teaching and learning advice contained in course arrangement documentation has 'been informed by research into successful teaching is not so evident', suggesting that the source of unease on this issue was a difference in outlook between believing policy makers and sceptical practising teachers and academics. Adding to problems during this period were teachers frustrations about the lack of feedback on each pupil's performance in national examinations, as it indicated a lack of sympathy and understanding about how assessment feedback could be incorporated into attempts to improve teaching, learning and assessment in future years.

These problems might have been less acute, if during the consultation phase for higher levels awards within the Higher Still programme, the teaching profession had committed itself to a more complete form of integrated teaching, learning and assessment, where performance and analytical competencies were recognised within the same outcome. However, this did not occur, mostly so that pupils whose main abilities were in performance could achieve a distinct 'unit' credit. However, this decision had worrying ramifications, as the integrated rationale no longer dovetailed with integrated assessment arrangements. Thus, the potential existed for the content knowledge associated with performance (often misguidedly referred to as theory) to be taught separately in detached class settings (Brewer, 2003; Thorburn, 2007a). Dispiritingly, Principal Assessor reporting for the Scottish Qualifications Authority (SQA) has highlighted on an annual basis the debilitating influence of rote teaching, learning and assessment procedures.

In analysing the main patterns of provision which were emerging nationally, Thorburn and Collins (2003) classified three 'types' of schools. Firstly there were 'trying' schools where the pressures of delivering courses were determining the quality of student learning experiences. Teachers were rather overwhelmed by the multiple challenges of attempting to deploy experiential teaching and learning methodologies, develop their own content knowledge base to cover adequately the width and depth of course information required as well as make effective curriculum decisions about how to complete assessment procedures. Thus, while teachers' beliefs were favourably disposed towards higher-level awards, for various pedagogical and operational reasons, teachers could not deploy policy as expected.

Secondly, there were 'rote' schools which were 'successful' in the reductive sense of the term. These schools had decided a priori that the extent of their assessment concerns merited the development of prescriptive answers which could be rote-learned by pupils. Consequently, many pupils were involved in 'elaborate charades designed to demonstrate progress at a systems level rather than in levels of learning' (Haywood and Hedge, 2005, p. 66). Teachers recognised the conflict that existed between their views of teaching when the course began relative to the assessment approaches which were in operation by the end of the course. Nevertheless, teachers considered it necessary to adopt 'set recipes' to try to secure high pass rates.

Thirdly, there were some 'successful' schools, where teaching was characterised by a high level of expertise in experiential methodologies, where feedback was effectively built into teaching and learning, and where the pupils were highly motivated and engaged with learning tasks. Pupils completed written assessment answers in the divergent open manner expected and were able to make informed and personalised connections between performance and the influences that shaped its development. Teachers in the 'succeeding' schools found that retaining a practical experiential approach was helped by their own self-initiated involvement in related professional development opportunities aimed at improving their content knowledge understanding.

Further research noted that these problems were not notably lessening with time. Thorburn and Collins (2006a) concluded that there is no compelling evidence, so far, that nationally the rationale for higher level awards can lead to high levels of authentic attainment on a sustained basis. Thus, the credibility issues which have so perplexed many in the physical education profession in their quest for academic recognition are only likely to be exacerbated further by this reporting. In explaining, the comparatively poor examination achievements of pupils, the major factor which emerged from teacher interviews was that the format of written assessment instruments was placing pupils at a disadvantage. Thorburn and Collins (2006b) compared oral and written assessment instruments and were not able to support this assertion. Instead, it was argued, that there was encouraging signs that oral assessment evidence could, in the continued absence of SQA feedback, provide teachers with information that could usefully be incorporated into effective curriculum decision-making.

The ongoing nature of the teaching, learning and assessment difficulties reported inevitably highlights a number of questions about the conceptual adequacy of arguing for practical experiential learning as the basis for trying to realise high levels of attainment within senior school examination awards. Some of these questions were explored by Reid (1996a; 1996b), but for the most part conceptually related arguments were based on an alternative conception of education which valued more highly practical rather than academic knowledge. In any event, these arguments were not discussed during the policy making process; evidence at the time of the disconnection which existed between the research and policy communities. In an attempt to produce a version of a higher level award, which could complement rather than contradict an academically informed curriculum justification, Thorburn (2008) argued that a greater focus on personalised learning through deploying phenomenological informed teaching and learning approaches would be beneficial.

The chain of challenges which presently exist, from the conceptual through to the operational, would benefit from a number of policy and professional development interventions designed to improve matters. However, due to limited local authority support, 'the lack of a professional association to voice its concerns' and the changing nature of HMIE remit, quite who is going to take responsibility remains of concern (Brewer, 2003, p. 592). This is especially so when further consultation on how the best features of Standard Grade and Intermediate awards within the Higher Still framework can articulate with extending the capacities of a CfE beyond the age of 14 are planned.

The changing fortunes of core physical education programmes

Despite the positive endorsement of physical activity contained in the Munn Report, the curriculum prominence of examination programmes raised concerns about the place and value of core physical education, where from the late 1970s to the turn of the century the time and priority afforded to programmes steadily decreased. Littlefield *et al.* (2003) found that in just under half of schools (43%), no provision was available for pupils in the senior secondary schools years (S5/S6) and in a small number of schools less than an hour of physical education was available in the lower secondary school (S1/S2) with no provision at all in the middle secondary school years (S3/S4). Some considered the prioritising of examination over core physical education was, in part, responsible for creating this problem (Cairney, 2004), yet the situation in Scotland reflects international evidence that core physical education programmes towards the end of the twentieth century were in crisis, as it was perceived to be remote from the needs of pupils and inflexible in terms of how curricula were constructed (Hardman and Marshall, 2000).

Achieving curriculum coherence for core programmes from the early 1990s onwards required articulation with the 5–14 national guidelines for Expressive Arts. The teaching and learning advice offered was particularly opaque for many specialist as well as for non-specialist teachers. The descriptive terminology used was heavily based on aesthetic references to 'space', 'dynamics' and 'relationships', and quite how this dovetailed with subsequent descriptions of outcomes, strands and attainment targets was a difficult mapping exercise for many teachers as they commenced curriculum planning. In addition, the national guidelines did not articulate closely with the rationale for examination awards, where as noted earlier, perceptual motor statements predominantly informed pupils' learning.

A decade later HMIE reporting on primary physical education indicated that only a third of schools were delivering very good programmes (HMIE, 2001). Weaknesses included a lack of specialist teachers – over 90% of physical education teachers are employed in secondary schools (Scottish Executive, 2005); limited professional development opportunities, limited integration with other areas of school learning and limited use of effective dialogue and diagnostic feedback. Overall, the emphasis on raising expectation led to a style of reporting that was more acerbic in tone than its earlier secondary school equivalent (SOED/HMIE, 1995).

Nevertheless, the security of having national guidelines for pupils aged 5–14 tended to highlight the curriculum weakness of core physical education programmes during the middle years of secondary schooling, for pupils aged 15 and 16. Relative to other areas of provision, physical education in these years has continued to be relatively unregulated and often squeezed for curriculum time by other competing priorities. The criticism emerging of low interest and participation rates (for girls in particular) along with concerns about the lack activity choices available to pupils made uncomfortable reading for the profession (Scottish Executive, 2004a). The influence of sport with its bias towards team games and a focus on winning combined with the overuse of narrow reproductive performance improvement pedagogical approaches have often been cited as major reasons why pupils become disengaged from physical education at this age. Within this type of sport-influenced environment, curricula have often consisted of compartmentalised activity blocks lasting a short number of weeks with little evidence of connective learning informing curriculum delivery (Penney et al., 2006). However, despite core physical education programmes being characterised until recently by such a range of concerns, the prominence of the subject has risen markedly during a period of recent curriculum renewal in Scotland. The next part of this chapter will consider the prospects which now exist in greater detail.

Physical education, health and well-being and a curriculum for excellence

The current policy emphasis is on achieving a 3-18 curriculum coherence with goals framed by intentions for pupils to become 'successful learners', 'confident individuals', 'effective contributors' and 'responsible citizens', with greater learning transfer occurring across the ages and stages of child development and between primary and secondary schools (Scottish Executive, 2004b). This process has been evolving since 2000 when the Scottish Parliament identified five national priorities for education, with a collective emphasis on improving equality and inclusion (Humes, 2003) and lifelong learning aspirations becoming the driver for generating educational improvements. Increased political interest and investment in education is matched by a policy of returning autonomy to teachers to exercise their decision-making responsibilities in trying to achieve generically framed educational aims.

The CfE policy emphasis has arisen due to concern about the subject-based bias in secondary schooling being of marginal value as the traditional arrangements for school certification have 'best served those who pursue subjects at university at the expense of learning for citizenry' (Humes and Bryce, 1999, p. 104). Within this type of curriculum, 'practical abilities, investigative skills, problem-solving, oral abilities and so forth got into the secondary curriculum, within subjects, but the strain they create for assessment and certification means they remain somewhat curtailed, indeed are under pressure to be reduced' (Bryce and Humes,1999b, p. 42). The historical tendency to innovate through subject-based approaches is to change within CfE as policy makers are now promoting support for increased curriculum flexibility and breadth.

The direct and positive endorsement of various Scottish Executive Health and Education Ministers has directly influenced the policy construction process as CfE contains a compulsory 'health and well-being mode ... (which) ... reflects new thinking about the strong links between well-being and learning' (Munro, 2006, p. 1). This enhanced policy position ensured that it became essential to legitimise physical education's contribution to a greater extent than previously as the subject 'is an area of the curriculum which, exceptionally, needs greater priority to support the health and well-being of young people in Scotland' (Scottish Executive, 2004c, p. 1). Thus, even though the overarching policy ambitions are for a de-cluttering of the curriculum and an increase in school-based decision-making, the politically-driven policy process has also insisted that the centrality of physical education to a balanced education is recognised for its health and well-being contribution and for its capacity to be the key influence in enacting the cultural change required. The predominant health focus arose out of concerns about low participation levels and the rapid increase in the number of overweight and obese children in Scotland over the past few decades. Moreover, the Scottish Health Survey (Scottish Executive, 2003b) reported that children's participation rates in physical activity were beginning to decline as early as age 4 for both boys and girls. This decline is much steeper for girls than boys, so much so that by the time girls reach their teens, only 35% achieve the recommended levels of physical activity.

In a policy sense, clarification about how terms such as 'participation levels', 'participation rates' and 'obesity challenges' are to be understood is clearly important, and these types of concerns dominated thinking on the 'Review Group on Physical Education' whose report (Scottish Executive, 2004a) discussed how physical education and school sport should respond to the interests and changing lifestyles of pupils. The Review Group was set up in response to a recommendation in the national strategy for physical activity (Scottish Executive, 2003a), which recognised the specialist nature of physical education and the need for high quality teaching, learning and curriculum frameworks as the basis for tackling problems with inactivity and lack of interest among pupils. The Review Group presented the case that all pupils needed physical education as the foundation for a physically active life. Moreover, to enhance social inclusion and engagement in learning, schools were considered as pivotal to the future of the subject as they are 'the only place where equity of access and opportunity to good quality' physical education programmes can be achieved (Scottish Executive, 2004a, p. 27). Within a short period of time core physical education had moved from a rather peripheral role, to occupying a position as the pivotal component of health and well-being, the 'new kid on the block' (Munro, 2006, p. 1) in curriculum terms.

The intention is that all pupils have access to quality physical education experiences throughout every stage of their school life and have the opportunity to develop the foundation for healthy and active lives. To achieve such goals teachers are challenged to change their pedagogical approaches and to view the contribution physical education can make with the widest possible lens, where courses achieve a multitude of aims based on a clearly articulated view of learning and where participation increases are sustained. Policy recommendations specify that the early education experiences of pupils should focus on basic movement skills and the links between physical activity, health and well-being, for without them 'pupils will be excluded from participation in many activities, or may find their enjoyment compromised' in later school years (Scottish Executive, 2004a, p. 27). In improving basic movement skills the difficult issue for policy makers to resolve was that if the focus on developing skills was pursued in reproductive teaching environments through familiar pedagogical practices, then it might make the achievement of broader cognitive, social and emotional development objectives more difficult to achieve.

In offering advice on curriculum planning the Review Group were 'convinced that extending choice beyond the traditional games' was the best approach for improving school programmes once basic skills had been developed (Scottish Executive, 2004a, p. 29). This position appears to have a degree of endorsement as recent HMIE (2008) pronouncements advise that there is considerable scope for physical education to fully contribute to the attainment of CfE aims by promoting in pupils a greater sense of responsibility and independence during their learning experiences and of increasing pupils' self-confidence and collaboration in learning. Yet, merely increasing choice might run the risk of modest benefits if pupils experience a series of 'learning to move' introductions to new activities relative to a 'moving to learn' informed curriculum, which more overtly addresses the lifelong learning priorities considered fundamental for longer term gains (Penney and Jess, 2004). Furthermore, the claim that pupils do not see the relevance of the more traditional curriculum activities appears open to conjecture. Scottish Independent schools have for many years delivered a 'traditional' curriculum which is dominated by team games, yet this does not appear to have a negative influence on the pupils' desire to take part voluntarily in physical activity (Littlefield et al., 2003). In addition, research has discovered that, from a physiological perspective, pupils currently work harder during games lessons in comparison with other activity lessons in the curriculum (Fairclough and Stratton, 2005).

The Chairman's Foreword in the Review Group report highlighted the difficulty there was in gaining consensus on a number of contested points, when it was recorded that many hours were spent in 'robust discussion of what is a very complex area' (Scottish Executive, 2004a, p. 3). The solution provided was to suggest that a mix of 'learning to move' and 'moving to learn' inputs was required. Overall, the types of discussion the Review Group members were involved with can be viewed as both a strength and a weakness of the policy process: a strength in that the wide ranging membership of the group ensured that the plurality of possible aims were explored, but also a weakness in that reaching agreement placed an excessive strain on achieving consensus within the policy community. In this environment, one risk is that the outcomes reached reflect a position 'that no party ideally wanted, intended or anticipated' (Green, 2008, p. 28), even though as happened with the Review Group report all members signed up to the final agreement; further evidence, if any were needed, that what matters in Scottish policy making is securing professional agreement. However, one adverse consequence of this position in the current context is that teachers can become compliant with a lack of policy guidance and interpret the mixed messages of policy reporting on subject purposes as an opportunity to continue repeating familiar curriculum content and pedagogical approaches which have been deployed for many years until greater clarity, leadership and direction is provided. In some senses, the problems of lack of engagement, which characterised physical education as part of the Expressive Arts in the early 1990s, could reappear when physical education is reclassified as part of health and wellbeing within CfE.

Consequently, the absence of a national steering group or equivalent organisation to monitor policy plans is surprising given the increased interest and investment in health and education. The implementation of policy appears to have adopted a relatively laissez-faire approach, which relies heavily on teachers to devise ways of meeting targets at unitary authority and school level. This could be problematic as planned improvements not only involve a re-conceptualisation of the subject, but the creation of new professional development opportunities which outline how pedagogically the teaching of physical education could become more informed and expert. In the light of these requirements a more robust and systematic monitoring of progress might have benefited teachers in schools as well as representatives of the wider policy community.

Additionally, greater policy definition about what precisely was meant by 'physical education' as opposed to 'physical activity' and / or 'sport' has often been required. In 2008, the then Schools Minister (Maureen Watt) ventured that the planned increased time allocation for physical education could be met by walking to and from school and through after school activities, a position which suffice to say would question the educational centrality of physical education and would likely inflame the views of many teachers. This perceived faux pas might well have contributed towards the Minister being replaced in February 2009. Nevertheless, the enhanced and exceptional level of political support for the Review Group report, which is reflected in the creation of 400 additional teacher posts and a policy pledge to provide two hours of physical education per week for all school age pupils, is largely seen as the 'biggest boost' to physical education in generations (Jess, 2004, p. 6). Accordingly, in the light of increased curriculum priority and financial investment, it is worth reviewing the challenges of addressing critical debates in physical education and analysing arguments for prioritising developmental programmes in physical education.

Critical debates in physical education

The Berlin World Summit on Physical Education in 1999 became instrumental in alerting governments of the need to implement policies which were based on high quality physical education programmes and which were supported by improved training opportunities for teachers (Hardman and Marshall, 2005). However, due to the short-term nature of many of the planned interventions, various authors have argued that the increased political prominence of physical education is not necessarily the same as a sustained commitment towards increasing the status and enhancing the educational worthiness of the subject (Kirk, 2006). Penney (2008, p. 37) has advised, for example, that for physical education to align itself with a remit based around reducing obesity rates and increasing physical activity levels 'may prove a costly sidetrack for the profession', who in any event might not be committed to the pragmatics of achieving such limited aims and in making a direct connection between levels of exercise and levels of obesity (Johns, 2005). Thus, there is a need for policy makers to avoid being 'drawn into the obesity vortex' (Gard, 2004, p. 76) and to recognise instead that to be properly physically educated involves being experienced in practical learning, which is filled with clear personal and educational relevance rather than being primarily involved in passively receiving teaching advice which is based instead on merely improving physical fitness and reducing obesity rates. Siedentop (2002, p. 372) has forthrightly argued that the core status problem of physical education needs to be directly addressed and comments that:

This, then, is the root problem – the direct study of sport skill and strategy through experiential learning is not considered to be of sufficient academic quality . . . Learning, basketball, volleyball, and gymnastics – and all the associated issues of training, technique, performance and strategy – are not worthy of formal academic credit . . . If we cannot confront that core problem, and somehow resolve it, then physical education in schools is doomed.

In summary, improved physical fitness, it is argued, should be more of an associated benefit of participation than a reason for participation in itself (Kretchmar, 2000).

Yet, policy makers might not agree with this view, preferring instead to believe that there is a clear link between poor physical health, increased child obesity rates and the ineffectiveness of physical education programmes in schools. For example, the only evidence presented in the Review Group report was health rather than educational evidence (Scottish Executive, 1998). Therefore, quite how to 'square the circle' on this issue is a difficult task and one which is added to by recognising that physical education is influenced by many contrasting and competing agendas; noteworthy among these is resolving issues about how the talent of particularly able pupils can be developed without 'compromising educational principles' (Lee, 2004, p. 8), especially at a time when preparations are under way for the hosting of the Olympic Games in 2012 in London and the Commonwealth Games in Glasgow in 2014.

The national strategy for improving physical activity contains frequent references to school physical education (Scottish Executive, 2003a) whereas the national sports strategy makes relatively few links between sport and education (Scottish Executive, 2007). Accordingly, the current policy position appears to be that it would be inadvisable and insincere to pursue sport-based strategies when there are such problems with the basic fitness and movement competence levels of so many school age pupils. However, as sporting success at national level has the capacity to increase nationalistic pride, it may be that further changes are planned. The SNP manifesto for the 2007 Scottish parliamentary election made a commitment to create six regionally based specialist sport academies with entry by application and ability. This innovation by itself would be something of a challenge to the entitlement for all principles at the heart of the Scottish comprehensive school, principles which are more obviously embedded within the three sports comprehensive schools operating in North Lanarkshire.

A further difficulty in years to come could be the extent to which it possible to articulate physical education with 'health and well-being' in a coherent and productive way. Some of the draft outcomes for CfE are framed around similar concepts and skills to those which were described for the earlier 5–14 national guidelines for the Expressive Arts (cooperation and competition and evaluating and appreciating). These proved problematic to implement in the 1990s and thus there is little reason to expect that they will be any easier to incorporate into curriculum planning now. Therefore, concerns exist, in the absence of more informed leadership, about how exactly teachers might manage their new curriculum remit. This is of concern, as Green (2000) found when exploring teachers' everyday 'philosophies'. Physical education teachers were often vague on how 'health' messages became integrated into their teaching. Additionally, Green and Lamb (2000) discovered that when 'health' became a permeating feature of the National Curriculum in England and Wales in the 1990s, there was no real change in terms of the activities which were taught or in the way they were taught. Teachers simply introduced blocks of fitness. Due to the dominant position of team games within the curriculum, fitness activities became geared towards improving fitness for games/performance, rather than promoting exercise for health and well-being.

Developmental programmes in physical education

With ambitions towards contributing to a transformative educational agenda, and of addressing some of the concerns sketched above, an important initiative in Scotland has been the recent designing of developmentally appropriate programmes of physical education. The programmes have largely been devised by staff from the University of Edinburgh (Jess and Collins, 2003). The original conception for this version of physical education was devised by two North American physical educators (Gallahue, 1982; Graham et al., 1980), whose work attempted to merge descriptions of established movement patterns with a constructivist-inclined pedagogical approach.

Encouraged by the general thrust of the conclusions of the Review Group report, a programme of developments are planned which would radically alter the content and teaching of the physical education curriculum, particularly in the primary and early secondary school years. Since 2001, an early years' programme 'Basic Moves' has been introduced as the first step in efforts to improve levels of movement competence, as it is this critical factor which is often cited in research as the main reason for high drop out rates in levels of adolescent physical activity (Jess and Collins, 2003). As 'Basic Moves' evolved, it has become the catalyst for numerous curriculum, pedagogical and professional development initiatives, which are informed by contemporary lifelong learning principles (Penney and Jess, 2004) and which recognise that lifelong physical activity is a choice activity and therefore understanding the reasons why pupils take part in physical activity is crucial in planning. The current priority is to design interventions which can indicate how core learning and authentic assessment practices can be delivered in an integrated rather than piecemeal fashion and which appeal to the interests of pupils.

Physical activity and youth sport

As well as fresh momentum for the centrality of physical education as part of health and well-being, there is a policy assumption that the benefits of physical activity and youth sport will become more prominent and embedded in the daily lives of pupils in and beyond school. Consequently, the Scottish Executive (Government) has invested in a plethora of programme initiatives to improve levels of participatory activity as well as identifying elite athletes. There is a further assumption with many of these interventions that the adverse effects of the acrimonious teachers' industrial action of the 1980s, which reduced a great deal of school and inter-school sport, can finally be overtaken with a more purposeful future beckoning. On both of these key assumptions, however, there appears to be considerable policy and practice difficulties to overcome if physical education is to meet policy expectations.

The first phase of the School Sport Coordinator Programme (SSCP) from 1999 to 2003 typically involved physical education teachers being released from their teaching duties on a one day per week basis to coordinate school-wide attempts to improve levels of sports-based participation. The first phase of the programme later became subsumed within the more overarching Active Schools programme. Evidence from the first stage review of the programme (Scottish Executive, 2007) indicates that despite the creation of 680 posts (more than half of whom worked as Active School Coordinators (ASC) in secondary schools) improvements in physical activity levels were modest. Secondary school age participation in 2005–6, as measured through analysis of participation rates in two local authorities, actually decreased by 9% with only 29% of pupils attending after schools clubs (Sport Scotland, 2008a). This was a poor response when referenced against National Strategy for Sport (Scottish Executive, 2003a) targets indicating that 85% of 13–17 year-old pupils are expected to participate in out of school hours sport each week.

Furthermore, establishing new partnership arrangements with the health and sporting communities was difficult at a time when ever more precisely defined teacher employment arrangements (Scottish Executive, 2001) and 'a heavily unionized workforce' (Ozga, 2005, p. 216) made developing a culture of extended school day volunteerism difficult to sustain.

In addition, the SSCP programme was not considered by teachers as a particularly worthwhile part of their professional remit or contributor towards career development. This may have been due to the perception that the remit of encouraging pupils to participate in and out of school was a lesser professional remit than that of a full teaching role. In any event, the SSCP remit at the time tended to be predominantly completed by part-time teachers who were available to take on additional employment, or by new teachers many of whom were in their first year of full time teaching. Evidence suggests that the participation and sporting supplements available were often lacking in lifelong progression with only relatively few examples of rich task learning providing transformative experiences for pupils (Coalter and Thorburn, 2003). Overall, this type of information provides an indication of how challenging it will be to equip pupils with the tools, motivation and opportunities to be more active throughout their school years and beyond. It also provides a Scottish-based reminder of an acknowledged problem within a politically driven policy process: namely that, national governments can gain kudos from the announcement of policy, but on the ground, improvements in schools and local communities remain much more difficult to detect (Lewin, 2005; Whitty, 2006).

Further policy interventions have tried to address the specific problems of girls' low level of active participation in secondary schools. The 'Fit for Girls' (FfG) programme was informed by two pilot initiatives (Girls in Sport and Physical Activity Project) which ran from 2005 to 2007 (Sport Scotland, 2008b). Initiatives in 27 schools showed that average participation rates increased from 18% to 27% in three-quarters of the schools involved. The FfG programme involved five trainers providing teachers and Schools Sport Coordinators with exemplification of how activities can be developed for girls both in school and outside the curriculum. Sport Scotland Board Member, and now Chair of Sport Scotland, Louise Martin applauded the programme as it encouraged girls to take ownership of their physical activity interests and enabled girls to choose a wider range of often non-competitive activities like dance and trampolining, as well as making the school environment more 'girl friendly' when it comes to physical activity. A noticeable feature of the

FfG reporting is the open criticism which was often made of physical education departments. For one school it was declared that 'There was neither an interest not targeted approach to improving girls' participation in PE and sport; consequently a recent school survey found 56% of girls were not enjoying PE' (Sport Scotland, 2008b, p. 18). In some respects it might have been expected that greater care would have prefaced this type of comment. For example, there is an apparent assumption here that lack of girls' enjoyment of physical education is linked to teachers' lack of interest and this might not necessarily be the case. For the present, this form of commentary highlights some of the challenges to definitions of professionalism which might exist when teachers begin working more frequently with a range of different professionals and volunteers.

In a crowded policy space it is also possible that various initiatives can rise to the surface in unexpected ways. Notable among these occurrences was the announcement from First Minister Jack McConnell in the latter days of the second Labour/Liberal Democrat coalition government of 2003–7 that competitive team games, both within the school curriculum and as part of the extended school day, were to become a component part of inspectorate review with HMIE only awarding top marks to schools which provided these opportunities. Due to the result of the 2007 national elections this manifesto pledge was never implemented, however the proposal is interesting to review briefly as it highlights how the policy process can be heavily influenced by a committed and interested politician as well as by the more standard routes of research evidence and/or traditional policy consensus. It also reveals that the short-term electoral nature of politics means that some policy initiatives can disappear just as quickly as they can appear. Furthermore, it also indicates that policy can be contradictory and confusing with, to some extent mixed messages emerging about the contrasting benefits of competitive and non-competitive sports occurring at the same time.

Outside of the traditional policy community, relative few groups have influenced policy in physical activity and school sport. One modest exception is the Scottish Schoolsport Federation (SSF). This relatively small organisation has quite skilfully used wider educational reporting outlets to declare its views about the limitations and missed opportunities of recent spending plans, where the links between physical education and school sport in the wider community have remained undeveloped relative to the situation apparent in England. As such, the SSF have been mainly involved in making principled criticism of policy plans and has been less involved in offering viable solutions to identified problems. In some respects, it might be necessary for pressure groups to try to build better connections with the Scottish Parliament through articulating more clearly not only what the perceived problems are but how they can be rectified.

Recently, it appears that policy has been influenced most by charitable organisations which are funded by private capital such as the Winning Scotland Foundation. The foundation aims to promote sport as the catalyst for developing positive thinking and for challenging Scots to fulfil their potential by institutionalising a culture of winning in schools. The Scottish Government and the Winning Foundation (previously the Scottish Institute of Sport Foundation) are in talks with local authorities to produce a motivational book to support the physical education curriculum in secondary schools (MacDonald, 2008). There may well be difficulties with this approach as teachers' traditionally high level of 'continuity and personal relationship within the policy community' (Menter *et al.*, 2004, p. 197) could become eroded as policy entrepreneurs seek through private funding to influence practice by working beyond the partially democratic boundaries of the typical policy community (Thorburn, 2009). In this setting, teachers might consider that their usual capacity for largely regulating their work has been to some extent compromised by new requirements to deliver materials which reflect a particular (and inevitable contested) point of view.

Specifically, with the range of ideas under review from the Winning Foundation there is some concern that proposals for greater competitive elite sport, as exemplified by the introduction of regional schools of sporting excellence and more afternoon competitive sport in schools (Coalter, *et al.* 2006), might not chime particularly well with many of the underpinning values of comprehensive schools: a model of schooling which has an enduring resonance with most people in Scotland (McCrone, 2003). Yet, as this example highlights specifically, there remains an assumption (as with increasing lifelong participation) that schools are pivotal to creating sustainable improvements, even though there is a lack of research which supports these assumptions (Wallhead and Buckworth, 2004).

More widely, the increased direct involvement of pressure groups, charitable organisations and national government agencies such as Sport Scotland, which is currently funded through the Department of Health and Communities rather than the Department of Education, highlights the tension which could occur with traditional guardians of the curriculum. Accordingly, quite how in future years stakeholders such as LTS, HMIE, SQA and the General

Teaching Council of Scotland seek to resolve any potential conflicts which might exist is likely to have a marked impact on the practice of physical education in and beyond schools.

SUMMARY

This chapter has attempted to review the nature and purposes of physical education by analysing official and unofficial views of physical education, and in so doing has made some specific comments about the introduction and development of examination awards in physical education, and about the changing fortunes of core physical education programmes, physical education, health and well-being and a curriculum for excellence and physical activity and youth sport.

Summarising developments in these areas within the context of examination awards, concern currently exists about who exactly is going to take responsibility for policy and practice issues which exist. There is a need for a range of professional updates for teachers which more clearly articulate how a philosophy of intention can be matched by a psychology of learning in ways which are clear, coherent and authentically achievable within most mainstream school settings. There is unease, as well, that the narrow focus on performance improvement might obscure a review of how physical education could respond to the range of opportunities which are available within the current policy context. Uppermost among concerns in this respect is how examination awards might be recast so that the best features of current awards can articulate with the agenda for health and well-being advanced within CfE.

While the introduction of examination awards generally added to the curriculum presence of physical education, core programmes have recently been characterised by lack of time, lack of progression and lack of curriculum priority, with problems often being most acute within primary schools. Yet the current policy context is now one which offers physical education the chance to address acknowledged barriers to progress, as politically the contribution of physical education has rarely been considered as being so central to the realisation of school and wider community lifelong learning aims. Therefore, physical education has the opportunity to recast itself as a subject that is responsive and sensitised to the here and now of political thinking and associated policy directives. However, political aspirations can change quickly and the policy making process requires to be continually critiqued in order to review whether progress is principled and well-founded in the longer term rather than just convenient in the shorter term. This remains a key point because, internationally, concerns about the educational potential of physical education has often been overtaken, both in terms of curriculum scope and pedagogically in terms of how learning is experienced by pupils, by the need to record short-term fitness improvements and/or meet activity target increases.

Nevertheless, there are some encouraging signs that after a particularly fallow period for professional debate some practitioners are beginning to seek out a more active professional role. For example, by the end of 2008, over 3,000 teachers have attended training sessions for Basic Moves and further support for developmental programme has come from the Scottish Executive commissioning the University of Edinburgh to develop and deliver a two-year postgraduate certificate in 3–14 physical education. In the first phase of the programme (from 2006–9) some 200 fully registered primary classroom teachers are developing a specialism in primary and early secondary school physical education, and with these teachers increasingly adopting leadership roles within their schools and local authorities, it creates for the first time a context for teaching physical education across the primary/secondary divide, which has so often in itself been a barrier to progress. In another development, 400 physical education teachers met for a national conference organised by Learning and Teaching Scotland (LTS). Collectively, these types of professional development are indicative of the research, policy and practice communities beginning to network more productively together.

Currently there is a policy expectation that improvements in physical education will dovetail with whole school initiatives and various out of school and community-based programmes. In many respects, this expanding area of provision is likely to raise challenges about how new working partnerships will become established in ways which recognise to a reasonable extent existing professional roles and boundaries. This might become important, not least in reaching agreement with new policy entrepreneurs who might wish to influence move overtly developments in physical education and youth sport.

Taken overall, analysis of the Scottish situation reveals a number of familiar policy problems. Uppermost among these is recognition that the outcomes policies are expected to achieve are often not delivered (Green, 2008). This is perhaps most evident, at present, in the way learning is experienced by pupils in examination awards and the limited return on investment which exists following attempts to created additional interest in out of school hours participation. Nevertheless emerging from this chapter as well are a number of opportunities which challenge the profession to 'seize the moment' (Thorburn, 2007b) and to make best advantage off the increased prioritising of physical education at this time. Therefore, quite how the profession responds pedagogically will be crucial for determining success or otherwise in future years. Accordingly, the next chapter focuses specifically on the pedagogical challenges of teaching physical education in the twenty-first century.

CHAPTER 3

Teaching Physical Education in the Twenty-First Century: Pedagogical Challenges

Synopsis

The aim of this chapter is to highlight the main pedagogical challenges teachers of physical education are faced with in light of the curriculum priorities discussed in the previous chapter. Overall, the chapter questions the idea that providing a broader curriculum will enhance participation levels in physical education, and suggests that more attention should be directed towards the development of teachers' pedagogical knowledge and practices in order to enhance pupils' learning experiences.

Introduction

Since the publication of CfE, there has been much policy repositioning in relation to the aims and objectives of physical education. The focus of this discourse has revolved around the idea that physical education should assume a dominant position in the Scottish Government's endeavours to improve the health of the nation. The purpose of this chapter is to introduce the notion that teachers' pedagogical practices may have a larger impact on pupils' participation patterns than widening their choice of activities. In raising these issues it is suggested that there must be a drive to better equip teachers to face the challenges presented by CfE and enhance pupils' learning experiences in physical education. Enhancing pupils' learning experiences within physical education, and adopting a 'moving to learn' and 'learning to move' informed practice, may facilitate the development of the skills necessary for lifelong learning and lifelong physical activity.

In order to explore these ideas, the following issues will be addressed:

- the physical education curriculum;
- participation in physical education;
- pupil-centred learning in physical education;
- current approaches to teaching physical education;
- teachers' beliefs about teaching;
- 'complex' theories of teaching and learning.

The physical education curriculum

Within a CfE, the outcomes for physical education are considered alongside those of physical activity and sport. They are subsumed under the heading of 'Heath and Well-Being' which also incorporates mental, emotional, social and physical well-being; planning for choices and changes; food and health; substance misuse; and relationships, sexual health and parenthood. The aims of 'Heath and Well-Being' are to develop knowledge and understanding, skills capabilities and attributes necessary for mental, emotional, social and physical well-being now and in the future. Physical education, sport and physical activity contribute to these aims by providing pupils with the concepts and skills necessary for a lifetime of physical activity. Consequently, physical education, sport and physical activity experiences should be broad and relevant, inspire and challenge. These ideas are closely linked to those from the physical education Review Group (Scottish Executive, 2004b). This group claims that pupils do not see the relevance of the more traditional curricular activities and recommends providing a broader curriculum with more choice. The Review Group believes that pupils will find physical education more meaningful and will, therefore, be more likely to continue to participate in physical activity during their school years and into adulthood.

However, one of the main concerns over the proposed changes to the physical education curriculum is that there appears to be an absent presence of discourse about *education* as the core function of physical education. Consequently, in satisfying public and political concern about the health and well-being of the nation, there is a shift in the way in which physical education is understood. It is important to recognise that physical education is more than the pursuit of health-promoting behaviours and attitudes. A key characteristic of physical education is that it can enhance pupil learning and development in the physical, cognitive and affective domains. For example, in order to access the physical activities presented to them within the physical education curriculum, pupils must develop their ability to perform a range of both simple and complex motor skills within highly dynamic environments. Moreover, the decisions that have to be made about the most appropriate skill to execute are cognitive in nature and are based on the pupils' knowledge about their learning contexts. Teachers can facilitate the development of this knowledge by encouraging pupils to apply skills such as critical thinking, problem solving, reflecting, observing and discussing. All of these are skills that contribute to pupil development within the cognitive domain and can transfer across a range of learning environments.

From an affective perspective, by encouraging pupils to listen, share and show commitment, engagement in learning activities in physical education can enhance pupils' value systems. Furthermore, by abiding by rules that are associated with concepts of right and wrong, activities within physical education afford pupils the opportunity to develop and express their moral values in the form of fairness, integrity, justice and in making judgements about foul play and cheating (Theodoulides and Armour, 2001). Importantly, the development of such affective competencies can result in pupils becoming more satisfied with their physical education experiences and enjoy physical education more, which may have 'implications for motivation and continued participation, even after schooling has been completed' (Holt et al., 2002, p. 167). By broadening the curriculum to include more lifetime activities, and by focussing more on health-related outcomes in physical education, teachers may give pupils the opportunity to sample activities such as skateboarding and yoga, but may not provide them with opportunities to explore each activity in a deep and rigorous way. This could have a negative impact on pupil learning within each domain.

Importantly, the claim that pupils do not see the relevance of the more traditional curricular activities is not underpinned by any empirical research. As alluded to in the previous chapter, Scottish Independent Schools are known to deliver a 'traditional' curriculum that is dominated by team games, yet this does not appear to have a negative influence on the pupils' participation in extracurricular physical education (Littlefield et al., 2003). Additionally, Gray et al. (2008) found pupils in schools in Scotland could relate to traditional activities such as hockey and rugby, and believed that they were an important part of the physical education curriculum. Those pupils who disliked traditional activities did so because of their low levels of perceived competence in those activities, not because they did not value them.

Participation in physical education

Perception of competence is particularly important in relation to pupils' participation in physical education because it has the capacity to increase their levels of intrinsic motivation. When young people are motivated to participate in physical education and physical activity, they are more likely to continue to participate (Weiss and Ferrer-Caja, 2000). Within the context of physical education, perception of competence usually refers to a belief about physical ability. It is developed as a function of previous mastery experiences and is enhanced by practice and teaching strategies such as feedback and modelling (Alderman, 2003). Not only is perceived competence a strong predictor of intrinsic motivation, it also influences subsequent motivated behaviours such as selecting challenging tasks, applying effort and persistence (Weiss and Ferrer-Caja, 2000). For example, Klint and Weiss (1987) found that children who were rated as high in perceived competence valued skill learning more than those with low perceived competence and were more willing to apply effort to increase their competence levels. Importantly, learning environments that facilitate improvements in performance and perceived competence also increase the likelihood that children will continue to participate in physical activity (Klint and Weiss, 1987).

A key consideration for teachers of physical education is that there is a difference between the ways in which younger children perceive their physical competence compared to adolescents (Xiang et al., 2001). This difference could go some way to explain why there is such a dramatic fall in participation levels as children in Scotland move from the primary sector into secondary school education (Scottish Executive, 2003a). Children in the early primary years have a limited cognitive capacity and are, therefore, unable to distinguish between effort and ability (Welk, 1999). This means that they evaluate their competence based on how much effort they apply to a task. However, as they develop, their cognitive capacity increases and they acquire a greater understanding of what it takes to improve their performance, for example, increasing task difficulty, sustained effort and use of learning strategies. They also become more able to evaluate their performance by comparing it to previous attempts, model performers and assessing the outcome of their performance. This knowledge makes it possible for them to form a connection between their perceived competence and their actual competence. Consequently, when pupils' performance improves, perceived competence increases. This is true even for adolescent girls who are known to be more likely to drop out of physical activity than adolescent boys. Equally, however, adolescents' increased cognitive capacity means that they are more able to recognise when their actual competence is poor. In many cases, this results in low levels of perceived competence, which can have a negative impact on motivation, willingness to apply effort to improve and willingness to continue to participate.

There has been some acknowledgement within Scottish education that many pupils have poor movement skills. Accordingly, as well as broadening the range of activities that are delivered within the curriculum, the Basic Moves programme now dominates early years' primary physical education in many schools. The intention of this programme is to provide teachers with the knowledge to develop pupils' performance of fundamental movements, and thus lay the foundations for a lifetime of physical activity. Although this appears to be a positive step towards improving pupils' movement competence, it may also be necessary for teachers and researchers to understand the learning processes that occur during key transition phases for pupils (for example, from early primary into middle primary). In the light of the cognitive changes that take place at this stage of development, it would appear important to understand ways in which pupils transfer their learning of basic movements in the early years to more complex activities as they move through primary school and into secondary school. Consequently, key to the success of professional development programmes such as Basic Moves is that they develop teachers' understanding of how movements and concepts are learned, as well as the theory that support this learning. These issues will be explored further in Chapter 4.

In addition to developing pupils' movement competence (and perception of competence), the extent to which they enjoy an activity can either positively or negatively affect their desire to participate in physical education and physical activity. Indeed, Welk (1999) found that enjoyment was one of the most commonly cited reasons for children's participation in physical activity. However, although this lends support to the idea that pupils should be offered more choice from a wider variety of activities within the physical education curriculum, enjoyment should not be the only foundation upon which to initiate curricular change. A physical education curriculum founded on enjoyment alone represents a shift from the pluralistic way in which physical education has been defined, and may not be able to attain the educational goals set out in a CfE.

Pupil-centred learning in physical education

Teachers' success in improving pupil learning is largely dependent upon the environment for learning, the teaching and learning strategies adopted, and the ways in which learning is organised (Scottish Executive, 2004a). HMIE (2008) provides more detail about the pedagogical issues physical education teachers should take account of in the delivery of CfE, particularly in facilitating the development of 'Successful Learners'. The two key themes that run through the proposed ideas are that teachers should use a range of different teaching approaches and promote pupil-centred learning. One of the problems with this advice is that it sends a mixed message to teachers about what constitutes good teaching: a variety of approaches or a focus on pupil-centred teaching strategies? Sicilia-Camacho and Brown (2008) suggest that teachers have frequently been advised to use a variety of teaching approaches, but in doing so, often fail to meet the needs of the learner. Additionally, many teachers simply use a variety of teaching styles to portray teaching effectiveness or they tend to gravitate towards a particular style that provides them with more control over the learning environment, for example, direct, teacher-centred styles (Sicilia-Camacho and Brown, 2008). This is problematic because such direct teaching styles are less effective in promoting autonomy in learning, which is in direct contrast to pupil-centred teaching approaches.

In order to promote autonomy in learning, both practitioners and researchers have advocated the application of pupil-centred approaches to teaching physical education. Penney and Chandler (2000), for example, suggest that pupil-centred teaching approaches have the potential to develop self-directed and self-inspired learning. Pupil-centred teaching approaches not only develop more autonomous learners, they also have a positive effect on important affective responses such as increased motivation and perception of competence. Weiss and Ferrer-Caja (2000), for example, found that when the physical education teacher focused on self-improvement and self-directed learning and evaluation, pupils viewed their ability more highly. Similarly, Fairclough (2003) found that pupils' perception of competence increased when the teacher set individually differentiated tasks and allowed students to work at an appropriate level of challenge.

When teachers set individually differentiated tasks, or encourage pupils to focus on their own improvements in performance, they are exhibiting teaching behaviours that are associated with a mastery motivational climate (Ames, 1992; Dweck and Leggett, 1988). Motivational climate is a situationally induced psychological environment that can influence the way in which a pupil approaches learning. There are two types of motivational climate, mastery and performance.

A mastery climate is when the teacher focuses on self-referenced improvement and effort and success is defined as improving one's personal best achievements. In contrast, a performance climate is created when the teacher encourages normative comparisons and pupils' success is judged in relation to the performance of others. Previous research has demonstrated that the creation of a mastery climate is related to adaptive motivational responses, such as a belief that success is due to effort, high satisfaction in learning, high intrinsic motivation, low boredom, choosing more challenging tasks and developing a positive attitude towards the activity (Carpenter and Morgan, 1999; Parish and Treasure, 2003). Conversely, perception of a performance climate is linked to maladaptive motivational responses such as the belief that success is the result of ability, choosing to perform in non-challenging tasks, low perception of ability and a negative attitude. Developing teachers' understanding of the ways in which they can create a mastery motivational climate within physical education, therefore, may increase pupils' intrinsic motivation and autonomy in learning, and holds more potential for the attainment of the pupil-centred aims of a CfE.

Unfortunately, direct teaching styles, which are linked to the creation of a performance motivational climate, still dominate teaching in Scotland and the UK (Capel, 2007; Morgan et al., 2005; Thorburn, 2007b). Gray (2008), for example, found that physical education teachers in both primary and secondary schools spoke about teaching team invasion games almost exclusively in relation to the development of motor skills. This was despite the fact that they discussed their beliefs about their physical education curricula in terms of health and enjoyment, and that team invasion games made a valuable contribution towards the physical education of their pupils through the development of skills such as problem solving, communicating and cooperating. Consequently, perhaps endeavours for change would be more fruitful if greater attention were to be paid to the development of teacher knowledge and practice through appropriate professional development programmes, rather than providing pupils with a broader curriculum and more choice. This is an issue that will be further explored in Chapter 4.

Current approaches to teaching physical education

Although HMIE reported in 1995 and 2001 that many instances of good practice were observed during physical education lessons, both reports also indicated that there were too many occasions where the teacher focused on the development of techniques at the expense of other areas of learning. Moreover, the 2001 report on primary physical education highlighted that teachers often taught basic motor skills out of the context of the activity, and that this resulted in pupil boredom and lack of motivation. This method of teaching reflects a traditional approach to teaching physical education that is both skill-focused and teacher-directed. The skills are usually practised through repetition and progressive tasks that move from closed to open situations, or part to whole skill performances. In this way, the pupils can focus on key technical components of the skill and replicate a model performance provided to them by the teacher (Williams and Hodges, 2005). The teacher facilitates this process by providing feedback to the pupils, feedback linked to predetermined technical components of the skill. Teachers teach in this way because they believe that pupils cannot access each activity successfully unless they are able to perform the skills of those activities first. However, one of the problems with this approach is that when the practice environment is detached from the activity, many pupils do not see the relevance, meaning or value in their actions. This means that pupils often find it difficult to transfer their previously 'learned' skills into the main activity, which usually results in increased errors in performance.

Teacher-directed approaches in physical education are also very demanding for the teacher because they are at the heart of the process, delivering the 'knowledge' that has to be 'learned'. Moreover, when the teacher takes control of the learning environment in this way, pupils often apply rote-learning strategies in order to memorise this knowledge. Rote learning may satisfy the pupils' and teacher's immediate needs, as has been evidenced in the delivery of Higher Still Physical Education (HSPE) (Thorburn and Collins, 2006), but is ineffective in the long-term construction of meaningful knowledge.

This traditional skills-first teaching approach is reflective of the reproductive teaching styles (Mosston and Ashworth, 2002). Mosston identified a range of eleven teaching styles based on a gradual shift of decisions from the teacher to the pupil. Furthermore, the styles vary according to their ability to encourage pupils to reproduce or produce knowledge. Within the reproductive cluster, the teacher makes the majority of the decisions and attempts to influence the ways in which the learner uses predetermined knowledge. Within the productive cluster, the pupils are encouraged to take responsibility for their own learning in order to discover 'new' knowledge (Mosston and Ashworth, 2002). Research into the use of Mosston's teaching styles supports the idea that teachers use the reproductive styles more than the productive styles because they believe that they are more effective in developing motor skills (Cothran *et al.*, 2005; Kulinna and Cothran, 2003). This strong belief about the importance of developing motor skills also means that when teachers are faced with a new curriculum to deliver, for example, one that focuses on the development of health-promoting behaviours and knowledge, this makes little impact on the way in which they teach. Accordingly, it is important that teachers in both primary and secondary schools in Scotland begin to question their own beliefs about teaching, and develop a broader view about physical education and physical education teaching. This may encourage them to alter their beliefs so that they are both willing and able to implement the pedagogical changes required to contribute to the development of the four capacities described in a CfE.

Teachers' beliefs about teaching

Developing teachers' teaching approaches, or encouraging teachers to change the way they teach, is not easy. Teachers' pedagogical practices are based on their personal beliefs about teaching, and these beliefs are extremely robust. Occupational Socialisation Theory has been used to explain why teachers have fixed beliefs about teaching (Lawson, 1986). Lawson defines occupational socialisation as 'all kinds of socialisation that initially influence persons to enter the field of physical education and later are responsible for their perceptions and actions as teacher educators and teachers' (p. 107). This socialisation process is responsible for the formation of beliefs about teaching, which in turn, strongly influence teaching behaviours. The most powerful beliefs that influence the way teachers teach are those that have been developed from a young age, for example, their own school experiences of physical education, teachers and coaches. Stroot (1996) found that physical education students had positive experiences in physical education and that their physical education teachers and coaches were role models for them, and that these experiences developed their understanding of what it meant to be a physical education teacher. Griffin and Combs (2000) found that these beliefs were deeply ingrained in student physical education teachers and that neither initial teacher education (ITE) programmes nor teaching experiences could change them. Indeed, ITE appears to have little influence over student teachers' beliefs about teaching although students' placement experiences can influence their beliefs when more experienced teachers encourage them to conform to the existing cultures within the school (McMahon and MacPhail, 2007). However, often these cultures serve to reinforce the beliefs that students have already formed about teaching. Accordingly, this highlights the extent of the current challenge involved in implementing new pedagogical ideas that hold potential for meeting the broader demands of a new curriculum.

For those involved in the professional development of teachers to influence the way teachers teach, it is important that they have a deep understanding of current practice. In order to develop this understanding, Tsangaridou (2006) highlights the need to shift the focus of attention away from teachers' behaviours and strategies, towards examining the beliefs that underpin the implementation of teacher behaviours and strategies. Additionally, as beliefs and practices are a mark of both the past and the present and influenced by their local context (Green, 2002a), they should be analysed within the wider social processes and constraints of everyday life (Green, 1998). Green (2002b) uses 'figurational sociology' to explain how physical education teachers construct their teaching beliefs or 'philosophies'. From this perspective, physical education teachers' beliefs and thoughts are not individual, independent of other individuals or groups (in the past as well as the present), but are viewed as a consequence of their interdependence with other people, groups and contexts. Thus, to investigate teachers' beliefs about physical education, it is necessary to explore more than just their immediate circumstances; teachers' past experiences and local context also must be examined. Only by uncovering, analysing and questioning these beliefs can teachers begin to change them, and their teaching practice.

Teachers' understanding of theory will also influence their pedagogical beliefs and practices. However, developing teachers' knowledge of teaching theory may prove to be difficult. Many teachers do not see the value in developing their understanding of theory and, instead, prefer to adopt a more practical approach to develop their pedagogical understanding (Capel, 2007). Moreover, many teachers value curriculum knowledge over pedagogical knowledge, believing that knowledge about teaching is fixed or static and is represented by a taken for granted set of unproblematic routines (Capel, 2007). Furthermore, this is reflected in the nature of the CPD courses that teachers both demand and value. Armour (2002), for example, found that teachers could not conceive of CPD initiatives beyond the development of sport-specific update courses. This suggests that teachers view their professional development as a process where pre-existing bodies of knowledge are acquired, and then conveyed to their pupils. Once again, this reflects and encourages direct teaching approaches, based on the assumption that there is knowledge 'out there' that can be transmitted and learned.

In Scotland, the difficulty of developing teachers' beliefs, pedagogy and pedagogical knowledge is augmented even further by the pressures placed upon them to develop their knowledge of curriculum content, particularly content linked to the HSPE curriculum (Thorburn, 2006). Brewer (2003) indicated that teachers' lack of content knowledge was affecting their confidence to teach HSPE and so there was an increased demand for resources that prescribed the content that was to be delivered. MacPhail (2004) also noted this problem suggesting that it may result in teaching that simply reproduces curriculum guidelines rather than producing or re-contextualising such guidelines, and often, in reproducing curriculum guidelines, more direct, teacher-centred teaching approaches are adopted. This issue was raised in the previous chapter in relation to the attempts of the Higher Still programme to introduce 'performance appreciation'. MacPhail (2007) found that teachers did not take advantage of the flexibility available and instead expressed a desire for a more prescriptive course. Additionally, teachers believed that the application of performance-led, integrated teaching and learning approaches recommended by the arrangements document were unrealistic (MacPhail, 2007).

This evidence highlights one of the key challenges for those responsible for teacher development in Scotland. In order to promote real change in physical education, learning and attitudes to lifelong participation in physical activity, teachers' beliefs about teaching have to be transformed. They have to be brought to the surface so that they can be analysed, questioned and challenged. Teachers should be given opportunities to test their beliefs about teaching against alternative teaching theories and ideas. When this happens, and teachers are presented with evidence that there are more effective teaching approaches at their disposal, then this may go some way to influence their beliefs, and ultimately, enhance their teaching. Chapter 4 discusses this issue further, suggesting that both the content and the design of CPD have to change so that teachers are provided with opportunities to develop their theoretical and pedagogical knowledge in an authentic and applied way.

'Complex' theories of teaching and learning

Most teachers who adopt a traditional, skill-focused and teacher-directed approach to teaching physical education view the teaching and learning process as a simple and linear process. They believe that their role is to assist learners directly and progressively in the internalisation of pre-existing external bodies of knowledge about how to perform specific skills. However, this view of teaching and learning ignores the wealth of knowledge and experiences the learner brings to the environment, and fails to recognise the way in which the learning environment can influence what and how learners develop their performance. Moreover, teaching and learning activities within the physical education curriculum are very complex. Learning to play team games such as hockey or basketball, for example, requires the acquisition of a number of cognitive and psychomotor skills that are applied within the context of a highly dynamic environment. Consequently, learning in physical education is supported by 'complex' theories of learning, for example, constructivism (Oslin and Mitchell, 2006) and situated learning (Kirk and Macphail, 2002), both of which emphasise the interactions of the learner within the environment in the construction of knowledge. In highlighting this more multifaceted view of learning, Light (2008) describes 'complexity theory'. It is based on the premise that, although there are different types of constructivism, they all revolve around three key tenets. Firstly, that learning is an ongoing process of adaptation shaped by the learner's experiences. Secondly, that cognition is both an individual process and a social process. Thirdly, it rejects objectivist views of learning that knowledge is an internal representation of an external reality and accepts that 'learning involves interpretation in which there is no pre-given external reality' (p. 28).

Both constructivism and situated learning theories have been used to explain the processes that underpin performance in physical education, and both highlight the need to view learning as context-dependent, where the interactive components within the learning situation all play an important role (Chow *et al.*, 2007). However, although they provide a useful explanation of how game knowledge is acquired, they do not provide adequate information in terms of how functional *movements* emerge during performance. Chow *et al.* (2007) refer to constraints theory to explain how the learning environment can be manipulated by the teacher to facilitate the development of coordinated and goal-directed movements. Like constructivism and situated learning, this theory supports the notion that human intentions are 'embodied' and constrained by a number of factors including mind, body, social and biological contexts (Davids *et al.*, 2007). However, constraints theory also proposes that movements emerge from the interaction of these constraints with the task (the equipment, rules and boundaries of the game) and the environment (the surface, weather, light). When teachers manipulate task constraints, set problem-solving tasks and apply questioning techniques during physical education lessons, pupils explore a variety of movement solutions to problems, rather than passively receive information about how to reduce errors in their performance (Chow *et al.*, 2007).

If teachers develop their understanding of learning so that they view it, not as a linear, but as a much more emergent, dynamic, interactive and complex process, then this may encourage them to adopt different teaching approaches that offer pupils a wider and more diverse range of experiences that hold more potential for learning (Light, 2008). The Basic Moves programme, which aims to develop fundamental movement skills in the early years of primary education, is based on this very idea: namely, that learning in physical education is dynamic, non-linear and emergent. Consequently, teachers and students who have experienced Basic Moves training, either as undergraduate students, postgraduate students or on CPD courses, are encouraged to present movement activities within a variety of different contexts in order to develop movement competencies which are both creative and adaptive. Importantly, the movements are not presented in a curriculum that consists of blocks of activity, which assumes that pupils learn activities in a logical, linear and progressive fashion. Instead, they are presented in a process-driven environment that reflects the chaos and non-linearity of learning. For example, in one lesson, pupils can be provided with various contexts which encourage them to explore different ways of travelling, or they can be provided with various contexts which demand different categories of movements: for example, running, throwing and catching. Importantly, pupils are at the centre of the learning process and there is awareness from both pupils and teachers that there will be a variety of different movement outcomes within each context, and that some outcomes will be more successful than others.

In relation to teaching swimming within the upper primary and/or secondary school contexts, teachers who adopt strategies that are underpinned by 'complex' theories of learning do not focus on the development of stroke technique by introducing parts of the stroke in isolation, and then joining each 'part' to form the whole stroke. Instead, they provide pupils with much richer and more cognitively challenging learning environments. They focus on how learning takes place and how they can assist in this learning. Teachers take into account the fact that each learner perceives the learning environment differently and, as such, are open to different learning outcomes as well as pupil mistakes. The aim for teachers is to provide opportunities during lessons for pupils to discuss and reflect on their experiences, thus reducing the gap between the mind and the action of the body (Light and Wallian, 2008). For example, teachers may ask their pupils to perform the breaststroke, with no leg-kick, and instead, place a buoyancy aid between their legs. This type of task encourages the learner to work out the most effective way of using their arms to move through the water. Light and Wallian (2008) explains the impact of this task from a constructivist perspective:

> This problem solving typically occurs at a non-conscious, embodied level that can be seen as the body thinking (Light and Fawns, 2001). It also offers a task in which the swimmer can adopt a state of mindfulness to reflection experiences during swimming (Varela *et al.*, 1991). Most swim coaches do not reflect on this experience, but this task does offer them the opportunity to take a student-centred approach by asking questions and encouraging discussion between coach and swimmer and/or between swimmers. (p394)

If applied successfully, and each individual exhibits some improvement in their swimming stroke, this can have a positive effect on the individual's motivation to learn, enjoyment and confidence in the water (Light and Wallian, 2008). Additionally, because swimming has been used as a vehicle for *learning*, the outcomes of this experience may influence continued participation, not just in swimming, but also in other activities where pupils understand what is takes to learn, that learning has occurred, and experience the affective rewards that learning in physical education can bring. Importantly, from a curriculum perspective, this pedagogy is consistent with the four capacities of a CfE in terms of promoting a greater sense of responsibility and independence during learning, and developing pupils' physical, cognitive and social capacities.

The broader range of outcomes that constructivist teaching appears to afford and the potential links to the aims of a CfE is also evidenced in the Sport Education model for physical education (Siedentop, 1994). This is a pupil-centred curriculum model that aims to provide pupils with a more authentic sport experiences. Within this model pupils learn to plan, manage and run their sports season as part of the PE programme. The teacher's role is one of facilitator rather than director of activity and pupils adopt the roles of coach, leader, official, administrator and manager as well as player/performer (Hastie, 2004). The season is presented during the initial physical education lesson and often lasts for a complete term. Pupils are selected into teams so that there is a mixture of ability levels and they adopt different roles, which are likely to include player/performer, coach, equipment manager, umpire and scorer. Formal competition plays a key role within this model, it gives the season its structure and meaning and is usually pre-arranged so that teams can organise practices around their matches. The focus of learning is on developing both individual and team performances which means that pupils have to be aware of not only the skills required for effective performance in games, but also the game rules, principles and tactics. Research investigating Sport Education programmes highlights positive outcomes such as the development of social skills (Hastie, 1996) and feelings of affiliation (Ennis, 1999). Additionally, Hastie (1998) found that girls enjoyed Sport Education because they were given equal opportunities to contribute in class as opposed to traditionally being overlooked.

Further examples of constructive teaching approaches that appear to support a broader view of physical education are Teaching Games for Understanding (TGfU) (Bunker and Thorpe, 1982) and the Tactical approach (Griffin et al., 1997). These are game-based approaches that focus on game understanding, and where movement is developed as a consequence of the opportunities pupils have to explore each game situation. Once again, the teacher has a less direct role in the learning process, employing strategies such as question and answer, modified game and problem-solving tasks, thus giving pupils more responsibility for their own learning.

TGfU evolved from concerns about the way games were being taught in schools. Pupils were leaving school knowing very little about games and having had very little success in playing them. The founders aimed to challenge traditional games' teaching by presenting a more tactical approach where understanding the game through games play is the goal, rather than the acquisition of sport-specific skills. With this approach, games are often simplified by replacing the more complex game-specific skills with catching and throwing skills. Games are also categorised (invasion, net and striking/fielding) to highlight the similarities between games in terms of their structure and objectives. Consequently, teachers become facilitators of game knowledge rather than facilitators of game-specific motor skills. Game-specific motor skills are introduced only after the learners have acquired the appropriate game knowledge. Additionally, improved game understanding not only makes skill learning more meaningful, but also contributes to the development of the learner's decision-making abilities (Hopper, 2002). Research into the effectiveness of TGfU has found that learners developed better tactical knowledge and decision-making on and off-the-ball, as well as increased enjoyment and intrinsic motivation when compared to more traditional skills-based approaches (Allison and Thorpe, 1997; Jones and Farrow, 1999; Turner and Martinek, 1999).

The aim of the tactical approach is to combine the acquisition of motor skills and cognitive skills, both on- and off-the-ball. In order to achieve this, teachers become facilitators of game knowledge and game-specific movements, unlike TGfU where there is less emphasis on the development of game-specific movements in the early stages of learning. The role of the teacher is to select the tactical problem that has to be addressed. The learner then has to develop understanding of the tactical problem and work out the most appropriate game-specific motor skills to solve the problem. These skills are developed through question, answer and active participation in the game or game-like activity. The teacher has a less direct role in the learning process and pupils are given more responsibility for their own learning.

The research that has been conducted to examine the impact these approaches have on pupils learning indicate that that they elicit greater improvements in game performance, decision-making, game knowledge and enjoyment when compare to traditional, skills-first teaching approaches (Dodds et al., 2001; Mitchell and Oslin, 1999). They also highlight the importance of context in learning (Rovegno et al., 2001) and suggest that pupils should learn skills within an authentic environment that encourages them to look for opportunities for appropriate actions, including actions off-the-ball. Off-the-ball learning is particularly important, because the majority of games play occurs off-the-ball (Blomqvist et al., 2005). Pupils, therefore, need to be made more aware of their performance off-the-ball, and the contributions that they can make to the game off-the-ball. This may encourage the player on-the-ball to distribute the ball more equitably (and appropriately) during game play, which could have a positive influence on pupils' involvement and confidence during the game. Ultimately, this will have implications for learning, especially in classes of mixed ability. Clearly, approaches such as TGfU and the curriculum model Sport Education have the potential to impact on learning in a broad and meaningful way, focusing on the individual pupil in order to enhance learning within the cognitive, affective and physical domains. Consequently, they appear to offer a means by which teachers in Scotland might attempt to reach the learning outcomes proposed by a CfE.

As highlighted earlier, there are some teachers who uphold a rather narrow view of physical education, adopting a position that focuses on the development of motor skills and games. This may be why game-based teaching approaches that take a more holistic approach to teaching games have yet to make any significant impact on the practice of teachers in schools in Scotland (Thorburn, 2007b). Capel (2000) suggests that this is because teachers are more familiar with technical approaches and are therefore more confident to teach this way. Supporting this view, Butler and McCahan (2005) noted that physical education teachers continue to use technical approaches because this is they way they were taught when they were pupils. Kirk (2005) claims that teachers may be resistant to TGfU because it exposes their lack of experience and game knowledge. In order to teach using game-based, tactical approaches teachers require an in-depth knowledge about effective performance, as well as the theory that underpins teaching and learning. Games are complex in nature and, for some teachers, developing such knowledge may not be easy. This may be why many teachers choose to adopt a much more low-risk approach to developing their own teaching performance.

To date, there is a dearth of research evidence to explain how teachers in schools in Scotland teach physical education, or why they teach in a particular way. It is important to investigate teachers' pedagogical practices in order to understanding the types of learning experiences they create for their pupils. This may provide valuable information for those responsible for ITE and teacher education/development with information that facilitates the development of teaching in Scotland and thus improvements in pupils' learning in physical education.

SUMMARY

The direction of physical education in the twenty-first century in Scotland appears to be changing. In an endeavour to contribute to improving the health and well-being of the nation, the aim for physical education in primary and secondary schools is to encourage individuals to pursue a physically active lifestyle (Bailey et al., 2008). A key assumption on which this change is founded is the notion that pupils are disengaged from physical education and physical activity because they cannot relate to the activities presented to them within the traditional curriculum. However, children become disengaged from, or uninterested in, physical education, not because of the activities themselves, but because of other factors such as perception of competence and enjoyment, factors that teachers can have some control over. The problem of inactivity amongst pupils, therefore, may be better addressed by focusing more attention on teacher development.

Although CfE aims to provide a more connected and coherent curriculum, as yet, it does little to provide those working in physical education with direction linked to their own views about the purposes of physical education. It is clear that there is a political drive to improve the health of the nation, and physical education can play a part in educating children about health issues. However, it is also important that, at such a critical time of change, there is more debate within the profession about the purposes of physical education. It is particularly important that teachers play a role in this debate since they are the ones responsible for the delivery of the physical education curriculum. They hold valuable knowledge about their pupils, the curriculum and resources, and this knowledge should be used to debate the future of physical education in Scotland. Their involvement will enable teachers to develop a more personal and well-informed perspective about the role of physical education. This is important because, ultimately, it will impact on what is taught and how it is taught. Debate within the profession may also be the catalyst that teachers need to boost their aspirations to improve their own teaching performance, something that is necessary if teachers are to be equipped with the skills and abilities required to interpret and implement CfE, even in the absence of a vision of physical education that looks beyond improving the health and well-being of children and young people.

The task for teachers, policy makers and those involved in teacher education is a great one, but a critical one. Working from a clear view of what physical education means, teachers should be encouraged to increase their understanding of the theoretical constructs that underpins their pedagogical practice (Capel, 2007; Light, 2008). They should understand that learning is a complex process, underpinned by theory, and that with this understanding they should aim to adopt teaching approaches that offer pupils a wider and more diverse range of experiences that will enhance their capacity for learning (Light, 2008). Understanding theory may also encourage teachers to question their current beliefs about teaching and to adopt alternative, more pupil-centred approaches so that they may enhance their pupils' learning and performance at the appropriate rate and level. This will impact positively on the affective responses that are critical to engagement and continued participation in physical education and physical activity (Li et al., 2007; Wigfield and Eccles, 2000) and ensure that the physical education curriculum is delivered in a way that makes a positive contribution to the health and well-being of children and adults in Scotland.

The following chapter aims to review the professionalism and professional development challenges that have been highlighted in Chapters 2 and 3. Against the backdrop of a new position for physical education, it aims to present ideas about the type of opportunities and experiences which it might be useful to include within initial teacher education and professional development programmes for experienced teachers. It also aims to identify the ways in which partnership with the health and sporting communities could be further developed.

CHAPTER 4

Professionalism and Professional Development

Synopsis

The aim of this chapter is to review the major professionalism and professional development challenges ahead in physical education. Following an introduction to the chapter, the types of opportunities and experiences it might be useful to include within initial teacher education and professional development programmes for experienced teachers are considered. This is followed by a review of how partnership approaches with the health and sporting communities could be further developed. These challenges are pertinent to explore given the new centrality of physical education curriculum and the policy expectation that programmes in schools can articulate with the benefits to society of improving lifelong physical activity and achieving greater sporting excellence. For these reasons, physical educationalists require to be alert to current professionalism debates and understanding of the future ways in which professional development opportunities might be provided.

Introduction

In 2007, there were 1,756 specialist teachers of physical education teaching in 378 state secondary schools (Scottish Government, 2008), an increase from 1,544 and 1,657 teachers in the two previous years. Overall, the numbers of teachers in post shows a steady increase, but one which is below the rate of increase expected following earlier policy commitments (Scottish Executive, 2004c). By contrast, the low level of primary provision remains. In 2007, there were only 154 specialist primary physical education teachers for 2,168 state primary schools. Across all subjects in secondary schools, the gendered nature of the teaching force continues with 60% of teachers being female.

However, provision is more equal in physical education (891 female teachers' vs 865 male teachers). The average physical education teacher is 40 years old, slightly younger than the norm for all secondary school teachers of 43.5 years (Scottish Government, 2008). Overall, the responsibilities for those involved in professional development remains a considerable one, given the increasing number of physical teachers in post and the continuing imbalance between primary and secondary school provision.

As noted in Chapter 2, during the early 1970s the focus of teachers' professionalism in physical education was mainly on subject-specific issues; for example, content knowledge of practical activities and effective teaching approaches. This, combined with a broad general overview of educational aims and a motivating and sympathetic presence, would largely equip teachers to manage their curriculum and whole school remit. Teaching, at the time, was relatively unencumbered in comparison with fulfilling the multiple agendas of the present day. Nowadays, there is an expectation that professional development can assist teachers in reflecting on their practice in seeking to improve their contribution to learning and whole school improvement, as well as an expectation that professional development measures will ensure that teachers' performance matches the latest accountability requirements of local authorities and HMIE (Boyd, 2005). Thus, improving professionalism is concerned with teachers' beliefs and values as well with questions about how the practice of physical education chimes with wider educational agendas and standards of national accountability.

Accordingly, as Chapters 2 and 3 have attempted to identify, there are now a large number of policy initiatives and pedagogical developments in physical education about which teachers are challenged to possess an informed opinion and up-to-date understanding. These include, for example, the ability to plan and deliver a range of examination as well as core programmes of physical education, to contribute towards improving primary school age physical education, to be capable of articulating the aims of physical education with whole school aims (e.g. through CfE and contemporary definitions of lifelong learning) and to consider the contribution of physical education in meeting the wider agendas of out of school physical activity and youth sport. Implicit as well in the descriptions above is a requirement that physical education teachers possess an informed understanding of social justice agendas, the nature of learning and the wider responsibilities of being a teacher in general.

So, quite how fulfilling this remit can be achieved requires review and, therefore, the focus of this chapter is on analysing the conceptual and implementation issues most associated with providing support for the key stages of professionalism detailed below. These are:

- initial teacher education programmes at undergraduate and postgraduate level;
- professional development programmes for experienced teachers;
- partnerships with the health and sporting communities.

Initial teacher education programmes at undergraduate and postgraduate level

Since the mid 1970s physical education teaching has been a graduate-only profession with the majority of current teachers having completed four-year undergraduate programmes. Provision for student teachers existed at Jordanhill College for men and Dunfermline College of Physical Education for women until the two institutions merged in 1986, with teacher education programmes continuing at the Dunfermline College campus in Cramond, Edinburgh. After joining Moray House School of Education in 1987 and becoming an overall part of Heriot-Watt University, a further change saw Moray House School of Education merge with the University of Edinburgh in 1999. The Cramond campus closed in 2001, and since then student teaching has taken place at the Moray House School of Education campus in central Edinburgh.

For at least a decade, undergraduate numbers in student teaching at Moray House have remained static, with around 100 student teachers in each year of the programme. This model of teacher education has an academic and professional focus with a progressive series of school placements being a central feature of each year of the course. This model is capable of carefully specifying standards and expectations and of providing a stable supply of future teachers. However, it is also a relatively expensive and inflexible model, as it requires a lot of lecturer contact time to service the course both in terms of teaching at Moray House and for completing placement visits to all parts of the country.

By comparison with the stability described above, there has recently been an expansion in the number and range of sport-related degrees programmes available in Scottish universities with nearly half (8 of the main 15 universities) offering undergraduate programmes in some form. Some of these can be used as the graduate entry point for one-year postgraduate physical education teaching programmes. Since 2004, programmes have begun at the University of Strathclyde, the University of Edinburgh and Paisley University. Numbers have been lower for programmes at postgraduate level, with around 60 student teachers per annum completing awards. From 2007, Stirling University have also begun offering four-year undergraduate programmes.

During the preparations for the introduction of postgraduate provision there was unease about the level of practical activity undergraduate students would have completed. The eventual agreement was to require applicants to possess a sport-related first degree which involved a significant amount of practical activity time. And, while the General Teaching Council for Scotland (GTCS) and HMIE will have some role in validating and monitoring degree programmes, it will predominantly be teacher education institutions which have the major responsibility in devising programmes that equip student teachers with the specialist subject knowledge and general understanding of teacher professionalism which is required. As student teachers spend approximately half of their 36-week postgraduate training in schools, success is likely to be highly dependent on the partnership arrangements which exist with placement schools.

Indeed, the challenge for all of the above programmes is how best to build effective partnership collaborations between university lecturers and school teachers at a time when achieving progress can be adversely rather than constructively influenced by the academic (research) intentions of universities relative to the professional (practitioner) priorities of schools. For example, a representative of the Scottish Local Authority Network of Physical Education recently commented that the undergraduate 'degree qualification sits around standards set by a university, not necessarily the employability of the student', with the major point of contention being that students require to 'pick up more of the physical side of the B.Ed qualification' when on school placement (Hepburn, 2009, p. 6). The current situation, therefore, is often one where there is divided opinion about how best to provide support for student teachers, and accordingly the remainder of this part of the chapter will review some of the most contested components of related discussions.

A starting point, which merits some attention in light of the importance of beliefs and values (Chapter 3) in shaping teachers' own definition of professionalism, is the question: What does joining a four-year undergraduate programmes reveal about potential applicants? Curtner-Smith and Meek (2000) outlined the relative narrow range of socialising influences which shape pupils interest in becoming physical education teachers, and it is difficult to anticipate this not being similar for undergraduate programmes in Scotland given that many pupils are making career defining decisions at a relatively young age. This might matter as careers develop, for as Menter (2008, p. 821) notes, 'the inherent conservatism of the teaching workforce' is frequently cited as one part of the problem is building effective academic and professional partnerships. Clearly, this situation would not be helped if student teachers were reluctant to consider critically research perspectives on education, preferring instead to limit their analysis to a narrower range of functional physical education concerns.

Therefore, the type of candidate entering teacher education may have a direct impact on the future of physical education and on the successful realisation of a CfE. Both undergraduate and postgraduate entry routes tend to attract students with a very strong sports background, which is often developed as a result of their experiences in physical education and reinforced by their extracurricular sports participation. This is likely to have a powerful effect on student teachers' beliefs about teaching. Thus, it could be argued that the longer four-year undergraduate programme represents the best opportunity teacher educators have to shape student teachers experiences and beliefs so that they develop a much broader view of physical education, and one which is more consistent with the aims of a CfE. However, as alluded to in the previous chapter, this may not be easy to achieve, with a change in the way programmes are delivered required if these aims are to be met. Furthermore, this task is even more problematic for postgraduate students as they might enter programmes with a narrower and more specialist sporting background which is often linked to sports science and/or a specific physical activity. This can conflict with the type of expertise it would be expected physical education teachers possess in relation to a CfE; even though some schools might welcome the fact that some new entrant teachers possess a narrower and deeper level of expertise in some areas of content knowledge such as examination awards, for example (Nutt and Clarke, 2002).

Acknowledging the mix of academic and professional demands required of teachers could be made more difficult if attempts are made to meet continually the diverse activity requirements specified within some definitions of physical education (Hepburn, 2009). Nevertheless, Green (2008) in summarising physical education in England (where there is a preponderance of postgraduate rather than undergraduate programmes) notes that there is an increase in the number of activities being offered in schools rather than an increase in the frequency of provision in a more familiar range of activities. This portrayal is matched by official reporting which indicates that on average 16 sports are taught to pupils during primary and secondary schooling

(DCMS/DfES, 2006). Expansion in width rather than depth of provision is signposted for Scotland as well (Scottish Executive, 2004b), where continuing to add to the range of activities offered rather than replacing existing traditional activities (most typically games) appears to be what is intended.

Yet, pursuing a strategy of trying in teacher education programmes to continually add to the width of activity-driven teaching carries the increasing risk of marginal learning gains if students teachers experience mere activity sampling rather than a coherent set of learning experiences which articulate with recent curriculum imperatives (Scottish Executive, 2004a) and lifelong learning priorities (Penney and Jess, 2004). Clearly, 'the subject must be more than a list of activities' (Capel, 2000, p. 209), and consequently there are many complex issues to analyse if physical education is to contribute towards a transformative educational agenda which is geared towards highlighting how pupils' critical engagement with practically-based experiential learning could challenge much of the 'docility-utility' of current schooling (Kirk, 2004, p. 200). As highlighted in Chapter 2, many authors have recently reasserted the need for physical educators to consider critically what is distinctive about physical education, and not to become deflected by wider politically-driven agendas, which are often based on the notion that physical education can compensate for deficiencies in health and sport provision (Evans, 2004). Overall, it might be merited for those advocates of continually increasing the range of activities available to pupils in schools to reflect on the longer term pedagogical and professional ramifications of espousing such a strategy.

For the present, however, the range of practical activities on offer in schools remains a contested issue, not least because of its likely impact upon student teachers' abilities to teach physical education effectively. This remains a forceful point of commentary from teachers in schools, who over recent years have become much more influential partners and contributors to the education of teachers and whose role is crucial in servicing the various undergraduate and postgraduate courses on offer. However, if further attempts are made to service a professional remit based on increased expertise in a broader range of practical activities, there is a need as well to consider the pragmatic pressures on teacher educators. For example, on the four-year undergraduate programme at the University of Edinburgh, student teachers spend just over a third (35%) of their course on placement. Furthermore, when at university there is a two-thirds / one-thirds focus on specialist physical education and general education courses. There is also a need to recognise the wider perspective that university lecturers in physical education are increasingly required to produce high quality internationally recognised research and this inevitably means that new appointees are much more likely to come from an academic rather than a professional (school teaching) background. Reviewed in this way, it is possible to identify how achieving teacher expertise in an ever increasing range of practical activities under these constraints is undeliverable without some new thinking on how best teacher education programmes can merge with longer term professional development plans. Yet, given that one recommendation in the McCrone Report (Scottish Executive, 2001) was that lecturers in teacher education should be required to update their professional knowledge with periodic spells of school teaching indicates the extent of the misunderstanding of role and remit which requires to be bridged.

How then might the situation be improved? One suggestion is that a commitment to the prevailing policy view of 'professionals in action' and of a lifetime of learning and reflection could be serviced by having greater differentiation in teacher education programmes. Thus, specifically, within the area of practical activities, student teachers with high levels of professionally relevant experience in some activities could use their time to improve weaker aspects of their personal profile. This type of initiative might become the seed for student teachers to begin to develop the types of self-start skills needed to continually seek out worthwhile learning experiences, both in and beyond those which are formally provided as part of their teacher education course. In this way, student teachers could begin to view teaching as an activist profession (Sachs, 2003) rather than a profession where definitions of professionalism are more inflexible.

Thinking along these lines will not only shape the types of physical activities student teachers are presented with, but also affect the ways in which those activities are presented. Gower and Capel (2004), for example, suggest that student teachers who have a strong background in team games may gain more from a course that focuses on the generic principles of games and the different ways in which games can be delivered. By contrast, those student teachers with limited experience in games would benefit more from developing a deeper understanding of each specific game. Developing such multi-dimensional and differentiated programmes increases the prospect of student teachers being confident in their teaching and of providing more accurate feedback. MacLean (2007), for example, found that student teachers' confidence to teach dance was enhanced when initial teacher education programmes provided learning opportunities that developed content knowledge for dance as well as knowledge about how pupils learn to dance.

Teacher education institutions can further enhance students' teaching skills by working closely with teacher mentors during placements to ensure that students are provided with opportunities to teach those activities which they have had limited experience to date. This process would benefit from teacher mentors who have a high level of expertise in those activities where pupils required additional support. It would also benefit from teacher mentors who have a broader range of teaching methodologies at their disposal, and who are able to use these in a reflective and adaptive way. This may even include those teaching methodologies that are inconsistent with their own common practices.

Furthermore, Wright *et al.* (2005) suggests that teacher educators should adopt strategies that are informed by more complex theories of learning, such as constructivism or situated learning, when delivering university-based courses. In this way, teacher educators can become the facilitators of knowledge rather than the transmitters of knowledge as evidenced by encouraging student teacher evaluations, discussions, reflections and problem-solving. Collectively, this type of approach provides student teachers with a deeper and more meaningful understanding of physical education, and the ways in which practical activities can be taught. For this to be effective requires that student teachers' prior knowledge and experiences are uncovered so that, if necessary, their beliefs about teaching can be deconstructed and new ones formed.

Many of the initiatives sketched above (individually researched and differentiated programmes, improved content knowledge understanding, closer relationships between lecturers in teacher education institutions and teacher mentors in schools and research on learning informing teacher education programmes) reflect the intentions of the Scottish Teachers for a New Era (STNE) scheme; an innovative programme currently being undertaken at the University of Aberdeen, which might well come to inform future arrangements for teacher education programmes. STNE is characterised by a social-constructivist, flexible and enquiring approach to student teacher learning, which challenges the view of 'teacher as technician' (or perhaps teacher of sampling activities in a physical education context) and some of the expectations which student teachers might possess as they begin their initial teacher education.

Professional development programmes for experienced teachers

In recent years meeting the professional development requirements of experienced teachers has seen a general shift from a provider-led to a school-led system, a process accelerated after 1995 when Scotland's 12 education authorities were replaced by 32 smaller unitary authorities most of whom could no longer support an advisory service. In this increasingly self-reliant environment there was an expectation that teachers could somehow match their teaching and learning to curriculum outcomes, for example, as was the case with the introduction of higher level examination awards in the mid 1990s. With some expectation of improvement in 2000, the first Education Bill to proceed through the Scottish Parliament increased the role of the GTCS in providing career development and detailed a new package of measures including the need for teachers to participate in 35 hours of recognised professional development each year and complete an annual professional review. Additionally, the opportunity was created for experienced subject teachers, who wished to continue a teaching career rather take on an additional school management or pastoral responsibilities, to join the Chartered Teacher programme. The modular programme conferred expert status by requiring teachers to complete either university-based courses in areas of formal learning or by demonstrating reflective evidence of teaching ability to the equivalent standard. However, for various reasons, most teachers have not as yet opted to join the Chartered Teacher programme with only just over one per cent of teachers (569 out of a teaching force of 52,970) completing programmes (Scottish Government, 2008).

On what basis, therefore, do the vast majority of teachers and senior school management staff currently decide on annual professional development plans? Purdon (2003) notes that the imperative for professional developments to articulate with the national priorities for education has often led to a standards-based approach with an emphasis on competences, target setting, quality indicators and so forth being deployed. This has frequently resulted in a 'cascade model' of delivery despite its limitations in recognising the situational specifics of different school contexts (Livingston and Robertson, 2001). Whether this form of provision best promotes notions of teachers becoming increasingly reflective about their practice is open to doubt, and thus concern about the adequacy of provision appears certain to increase, given the teacher autonomy focus at the heart of CfE and the implications this contains for programmes of professional development.

By contrast to the cascade model of delivery, Kennedy (2008, p. 843) praises the development of the 'Assessment is for Learning' (AifL) programme; a national whole school initiative designed to improve the quality of pupils' formative feedback, as an example of 'research-informed teaching and collaborative working in ways which teachers feel comfortable with', as it allows teachers to make decisions based directly on the needs of their pupils. Considered in this way, it might well be that the secret of ensuring that experienced teachers continue to add to their expertise through reflecting on practice is best encouraged by providing them with opportunities for the academic world of research to merge feasibly with the professional world of school teaching. With these types of aspirations in mind, the next part of the chapter reviews three current policy and pedagogy contexts where it will be important for experienced teachers to continue developing their expertise in future years. These are:

- professional development within primary physical education;
- Curriculum for Excellence;
- examinations in physical education.

Professional development within primary physical education

As briefly outlined in Chapter 2, the low level of provision, specialist subject teaching and professional development opportunities have held back developments within primary physical education for many years. However, more recently, there are signs of the research, policy and practice communities working more constructively together to improve the content and delivery of curriculum. The general thrust of the conclusions of the Review Group report (Scottish Executive, 2004a) support the notion of revising the curriculum and enhancing the professional development prospects of primary school teachers.

Conceptually, the curriculum intention is that learning experiences will develop pupils' technical ability as well as the adaptability and creativity needed to successfully apply movements in increasingly complex situations. In researching the theoretical perspectives underpinning this form of learning, staff from the University of Edinburgh have recently been engaging with ideas from a range of different contemporary learning approaches; most notably social constructivism, ecological motor development and dynamical systems. Social constructivist and complexity learning theories propose that learning occurs in an active way where 'pupils and teachers together create, share and shape their own and each other's meanings' (Morrison, 2008, p. 27). The ecological motor development and dynamical systems approach declares that pupils learn to move their bodies in non-linear ways through exploration and discovery rather than in a pre-programmed way (Thelen and Smith, 1994).

Appreciation of these perspectives has lead to a gradual change in emphasis from a focus on the more traditional, behaviourist ideas of relatively definite technical forms of mature movement patterns to more complex notions of self-organisation and emergence, which recognise the different ways in which pupils move and learn. In supporting this process, various authors have advised that learning needs to involve 'dynamic, unpredictable, and even chaotic' behaviours and practices (Light, 2008, p. 30). This non-linear view of learning is also consistent with the teaching methodologies described in Chapter 3. Collectively, these views support the notion that there is the potential to deliver a much more consistent message about learning throughout the curriculum from age 3 to 18 through adopting constructive teaching approaches which enable pupils to develop skills and knowledge in a more progressive way which increases their autonomy in learning.

For these learning gains to become an established part of practice, teachers need to be creative and adaptable in their pedagogy, as there are no set methods or linear models of teaching delivery to follow. This is not a simple measure and is likely to be positively influenced by the provision of appropriate professional development programmes which address critical questions and search for ways to change existing pedagogy practices. Accordingly, the essence of the piloting approach adopted for developmental programmes under way is to involve academics and teachers in a combination of off-site learning and in-school experimentation and through the creation of a number of localised learning 'communities of practice' projects which were developed following discussions with local authority managers and the training of tutors who deliver courses and who offer follow-up support. This appears to be exactly the sort of intervention the Sutherland Report (1997), which provided the initial recommendations for establishing a national framework of professional development, had in mind as it contains the capacity to overcome the adoption of a rather managerial and overly prescriptive approach to professional development. The intention in the longer term is that these collaborative leadership structures can continue to support sustainable learning communities.

Curriculum for Excellence

Similar intentions to those outlined above might benefit CfE, where there is a need to recognise that the increase in teacher autonomy requires 'a shift in culture in how teachers expect, and are expected, to account for their professional development' (Kennedy, 2008, p. 843). In short, achieving a mix of teacher autonomy and a wider professional collegiality might be more difficult to realise through a managerial centred 'top-down standards' based approach to professional development. However, it may well be that a contrasting 'bottom-up' model of curriculum development would also have difficulty in coping with the scale of the demands associated with CfE, especially at a time when teachers may have become comfortable and to some extent reliant on being furnished with curriculum resources from stakeholders such as LTS and private publishers. Clearly, improvements in how professional development opportunities are presented to teachers is important and the type of initiative mentioned in Chapter 2, where over 400 physical education teachers met in 2007 for an annual conference highlights in the first instance the possible benefits of an awareness-raising event in signposting future professional challenges.

Thereafter, Armour and Yelling (2004) advocate that a focus on pupil learning and on teachers' everyday needs should form the essence of professional development opportunities with problem-solving tasks, collaborations, reflection and evaluation characterising delivery. In line with these principles, Tsangaridou (2008) suggests that development programmes should provide teachers with an understanding of theory about teaching which encourages teachers to develop their pedagogical knowledge. This would enhance teachers' evaluative and reflective skills, so that they can become much more adept at identifying their own strengths and weaknesses and the overall effectiveness of the decisions which are made during lessons. These ideas imply that teachers should consider auditing their current teaching plans and mapping it against the new expectations of the health and well-being outcomes within CfE and thereafter devising revised learning contexts with an emphasis on pupil-centred learning through problem-solving tasks. For example, it appears likely under the outcomes which are scheduled for 'physical education, physical activity and sport' in CfE that previously- mentioned initiatives (e.g. TGfU and Sport Education in Chapter 3) could become incorporated into the curriculum in ways which are principled and well founded and which overtake the 'root problem' (Siedentop, 2002, p. 372) of superficial learning and lack of curriculum seriousness which have surrounded physical education for many years.

Examinations in physical education

Following a review of policy implementation in Chapter 2, it is apparent that for experienced teachers three areas of practice require further professional support. These are, firstly, how can teachers' content knowledge understanding of performance-related concepts be improved? Secondly, how can the methodologies advised in policy guidelines be more effectively and authentically deployed? Thirdly, how can feedback from the assessment process inform improved teaching and learning?

Brewer (2003, p. 589) highlighted the adverse effects of teachers' lack of content knowledge expertise when stating that 'the extended advice regarding the nature of knowledge and understanding underpinning HSPE began to threaten teacher confidence to deliver the appropriate detail of required content'. And, while a top-down cascade model of professional development might work where simple dissemination of information is required, it appears less beneficial when a deeper pedagogical or professional transformation is required. From the findings of earlier discussions, which highlighted that the major type of professional development desired by teachers was for practical-based sessions which were immediately relevant and applicable (Armour and Yelling, 2004), it is clear that the dilemma which exists at present is how can this form of intervention be substantial enough to address the ongoing imbalance in attainment between performance and analytical abilities (Thorburn and Collins, 2006a). What appears necessary to include is some form of theoretical lecturer and/or teacher input which accompanies practical sessions and which explains feasible approaches for linking content knowledge with experiential learning approaches. These beginnings could attempt to sow the seeds for the longer term reflective practice ideas associated with the development of pedagogical content knowledge (Shulman, 1987). Van Driel *et al.* (1998) support such ideas and found that a cycle of workshop–application–workshop encouraged teachers to discuss, reflect, apply and evaluate different ideas about teaching. This resulted in gradual changes in practice, with an increased focus on pupil learning.

This form of professional development intervention would appear to be helpful as well in highlighting how the methodologies advised for examination awards could be put into practice in the manner intended. Furthermore, blending content knowledge with experiential learning would appear to have the capacity to reflect AifL learning aims, where feedback on learning experiences is used as the basis for teachers' discussion with pupils. This approach has proved relatively successful in encouraging teachers 'to engage with ideas, with theory and with principles' (Boyd, 2008, p. 432) and in closing the gap between their pupils' desired goals and present states of knowledge. Thus, linking this whole school intervention with the specifics of examination awards in physical education might help improve the ways in which teaching and learning is enacted. This could lead to an increase in practical learning environments as the basis for the development of related discussions, with all the improvements this might yield for the later construction of individually different answers that are true and authentic to pupils' lived experiences.

In reviewing, finally, how feedback from the assessment process can inform improved teaching and learning, it is apparent that changes in professional practice are required so that reliance upon external assessment results does not continue to affect adversely the quality of some pupils' learning and assessment experience. At present, it appears inconsistent of teachers to complain about the lack of feedback provided by the SQA without making better use of school-based internal assessments compiled during the school year and used as the basis for estimating pupils' end-of-course examination performance. Hayward and Hedge (2005) note the dilemmas caused by a profession which does not want a model of teaching and assessment, which has a high degree of reliance on school-based formative assessment, but then seeks the very type of information on learning which such assessment evidence provides.

In supporting teachers to make the three improvements necessary, it could be that in order to genuinely transform practice, 'a more sophisticated understanding of the interrelationships between research, policy and practice is required' (Hayward and Hedge, 2005, p. 69). If more than complying and reacting to the official policy position is sought, it might be that teacher education institutions (whose influence on policy has been modest for many years) could, given the increasing size and number of higher education departments within Scotland, be well placed to provide professional development opportunities for teachers. This appears a real possibility given the increased research role of physical education lecturers across Scotland. In this setting, the complexities associated with mastering practical experiential learning could be forthrightly addressed through interventions which ideally would meet short-term curriculum needs as well as longer-term professional development priorities.

Partnerships with the health and sport communities

As highlighted in Chapter 2, central government interest in curriculum developments in health and well-being have been matched by a similar determination to address the lack of sporting progress at both participatory and elite performer levels. In striving to improve matters there have been difficulties in persuading teachers to volunteer their time for leading and organising participation-based sessions (Coalter and Thorburn, 2003). Furthermore, the lack of primary age physical education has been a major limitation in trying to develop performance sport (Coalter *et al.*, 2006). Clearly, how physical education teachers manage their remit at a time of 'both opportunity and dilemma' (Brewer, 2008, p. 549) has implications for the future professional role of teachers as well as the practice of physical education. Consequently, the next part of the chapter explores two of the most critical challenges which currently present themselves within and beyond the formal school day. These are how to:

- work with other professionals;
- review attempts to improve provision in physical education and youth sport.

Working with other professionals

As noted in Chapter 2, the first phase of the SSCP was not considered by teachers as a particularly important part of their professional remit. Consequently the position was often filled by part-time teachers or new entrants to teaching. Further analysis reveals that over three-quarters of coordinators (77%) had difficulty in recruiting teachers to assist with the programme with only one-third of teachers (33%) described as being 'good' at volunteering their time. By contrast, the specific contribution of physical education teachers was greater, with two-thirds (67%) being 'good' at volunteering their time. The reasons for lack of volunteerism were variously given as an ageing teaching profession, lack of interest, lack of payment and perhaps, most significantly, by a desire by teachers to adhere to the new conditions of service agreement (Coalter and Thorburn, 2003).

The differences in levels of volunteerism are important, not least because historically the physical education profession has often been filled with unease over its perceived lowly status within an education system which has a bias towards 'education of the mind' over 'education of the body' (Armour and Jones, 1998). If teachers' extended school day responsibilities had been specifically addressed when conditions of service where reviewed (Scottish Executive, 2001) it might have been helpful, especially as the review was intended as a 'comprehensive and radical programme to help build the profession as a basis for giving it the trust and freedoms that are necessary in schools' (Peacock, 2004). However, as well as reviewing the professional construct of the modern teacher, the review was also required to acknowledge the 40% retirement rate of teachers expected nationally between 2004 and 2014 and the need to recruit many new teachers (Donn, 2008). As such, the review focused on the pragmatics of salaries, promotion arrangements, professional development opportunities and conditions of service. In this setting, it was perhaps inevitable that the opportunity to drive through reforms which had the potential to support extended school day participation in sport and many other activities was never really explored as, politically, there was a greater need not to become deflected from what were considered to be more pressing concerns.

Accordingly, what has emerged in subsequent years is agreement on teachers' role and responsibilities within schools, for example, where every teacher has a health and well-being, literacy and numeracy remit under CfE, but where definition on wider out of school roles and responsibilities remains unclear. For many physical education teachers this creates a dilemma in that enthusiasm to volunteer time could in some ways continue to exacerbate the status anxieties which have so exercised the profession over many years. Yet, to not volunteer appears to curtail the clear connections between enjoyment and participation in sport that appear so natural and which have so positively influenced many teachers in joining the profession in the first place.

In the absence of a conditions of service agreement which required all teachers to contribute in some way to the extended school day, progress has been more evident in other areas of policy. These have included the creation of Health Promoting Schools (Scottish Executive, 2004c) and the national strategy for physical activity (Sport Scotland, 2003) which details plans to increase activity levels over the next 20 years. Physical education has also been identified as a strong contributory part of the 'Active Schools' programme (Scottish Executive, 2003c); a programme which expects primary and secondary schools to work more closely with related education and sport communities in future years. Instrumental to delivering Active Schools is the staffing network of coordinators in primary and secondary schools across all of Scotland's 32 local unitary authorities (Sport Scotland, 2008a). As Brewer (2003, p. 591) notes, 'the lobby for sport, in alliance with claims being made for its benefits to health and as a vehicle for more socially inclusive practices, is having something of a political moment'. However, quite how this 'moment' will be grasped requires some further review. For while the present period is one where teachers are being urged to adapt and network more closely with professionals in the wider education and sporting communities in open, positive and constructive ways (Thorburn, 2005), it is notable that the entry requirements to become a coordinator are to be degree educated but not necessarily teacher educated. For physical education teachers, who predominantly completed the SSCP remit in the pilot for the 'Active Schools' programme, this could have contrasting effects. Some might consider it beneficial in having new coordinators in schools as it leaves physical education teachers free to volunteer their time as they wish. However, it could also be viewed as a threat if coordination remits began to impinge on professional areas which have, in the past at least, been considered as part of the domain of physical education departments. This could occur, for example, if coordinators became increasingly responsible for the management of practical facilities.

Of further concern are issues about how programmes like Active Schools, which are typically funded in four-year cycles, can become self sustaining. Coalter and Thorburn (2003) highlighted that there was no apparent exit strategy for the SSCP and this problem appears to be ongoing. Analysis of the Active Schools programme by an independent consultative group – the 'Loughborough Partnership' – indicated that there was much still to do, with lack of time (one day a week) for coordinators in secondary schools and the ongoing lack of secondary school teachers' volunteering their time being the biggest barriers to sustainable success. Thus, while the decision in December 2007 to continue funding at current levels for a further cycle until 2011 offers some short-term stability, it must be doubtful when faced with a severe economic downturn whether such high levels of financial support can be continued in the longer term. In this situation, it could well be that the relatively short-term investment in building better local partnerships between schools and the communities will achieve relatively little in the way of longer-term gains.

Reviewing attempts to improve provision in physical education and youth sport

What might help professionals in future years in making more targeted interventions is if teachers and coordinators alike could be as proactive as possible in reviewing the complexities which appear to influence pupils and young peoples' interests in physical education, active participation and youth sport.

By questioning some of the assumptions which are often made and thereafter trying to shape rather than to react to policy might be the most professional and strategic course to follow in retaining the current policy prominence of physical education and youth sport.

Evidence from the initial phase of the SSCP makes disappointing reading in this respect. Coalter and Thorburn (2003) found that in making decisions about the nature of the programme offered that over four-fifths (85%) of co-ordinators made decisions based on existing staff expertise, over two-thirds (72%) made decisions based on personal judgement, with just less than half (49%) surveying pupil opinions and just over a third (36%) meeting with pupils. Only 1 in 20 coordinators (5%) decided on programme opportunities in response to pupils' requests. The reported difficulty was that coordinators felt uneasy in discussing and responding to pupils' requests, many of which were undeliverable due to lack of facilities or staff expertise. Skateboarding was one activity which was often requested, but where demand was unable to be satisfied. In apparent sympathy with pupils' opinion, the Review Group (Scottish Executive, 2004a, p. 29) considered that providing 'more contemporary activities such as martial arts, yoga, dance, skateboarding and flag football could do much to increase participation'. However, while it might be easy to cast coordinators as rather unresponsive, inflexible and conservative, analysis also requires acknowledgement that facility and expertise issues and associated concerns about safety are highly likely to influence whether an expansion in provision occurs or not. In this respect, it could be argued that creating a community of coordinators should not be allowed to mask the generally under-resourced arrangements for community sport which exist nationally. Therefore, coordinators by themselves cannot be quite the panacea for all ills which is sometimes expected. Furthermore, it should not go unrecorded that while public and private partnerships building arrangements have led to considerable school upgrading in recent years, these benefits have not always applied to physical education and youth sport where many schools have lost the use of swimming pools and other facilities. For example, one delegate at a recent conference which explored ways of improving participation rates was dismayed that no swimming pools are planned for any of the six new secondary schools due to be built within one local authority (Hepburn, 2009).

Furthermore, it is important that the quality of provision is considered every bit as much as the nature of provision. In this respect, it would be useful in promoting links between schools and the wider community, if coordinators could develop effective working relationship with a range of local authority stakeholders in youth sport. Coalter and Thorburn (2003) found that coordinators valued the contribution made by youth development officers and coaches as they shared similar aims and professional practices. However, coaches' emphasis on enhancing sports performance may lead some pupils to believe that extracurricular physical activity is the reserve of the more able performer. Accordingly, the participation opportunities provided often might attract the more able pupils and exclude the least able. Therefore, a much broader and more pupil-centred view of teaching and learning might be required if pupils are to be given equal opportunities to participate in physical education and after school sport, even if this is in those activities which are usually perceived to be reserved for more able performers. Clearly, how the relationship between physical activity and sport is explained and understood by pupils is important. The inclusive model for physical education and sport created by Murdoch (1990) aims to meet the needs of all pupils through adhering to four key principles: partnerships between those involved at all levels of performance, the widespread use of modified games and sports, the provision of quality teacher and coach education programmes, and coordination of all aspects of policy development. Deploying models such as this might represent a feasible approach for increasing activity levels for all ability levels and interest groups.

In addition to generating improvements in the way professional communities work together, there is a need on the basis of decreasing levels of participation in school clubs in secondary schools (Sport Scotland, 2008a), for a more fundamental analysis of pupils' motivation and interest in physical activity. Put simply, it appears problematic to consider that pupils' interest in participation and youth sport is simply lying dormant and waiting to be released through the interventions of teachers, coordinators and development officers. Green (2008, p. 119) notes that the present time is defined by a 'broadening and diversification' of pupil interest with an increasing emphasis on the pursuit of 'lifestyle activities', which are characterised by being flexible and informally arranged and frequently based on activities that are non-competitive in nature. However, this increase in interest has not replaced interest in competitive team games, but has rather been added to the range of participation opportunities pupils might be interested in. Therefore, there is evidence that pupils often relish the perseverance and challenge aspects of competitive sport as well as the informality of flexibly arranged recreational participation. Thus, the profile of pupil interest which exists is rarely as simple as an 'either/or' decision when it comes to discussing the merits of competitive games vs recreational activities.

Consequently, experimentation in programme planning which is informed, in part, by discussions with pupils and which aims to develop school-by-school solutions that serve the majority of pupils well in their local communities appears necessary. In this respect, we would argue that some of the interventions discussed in Chapter 3 (TGfU, tactical games teaching and Sport Education) are worthy of consideration in more Scottish schools than is the case at present. Seeking to pursue qualitative improvements in these types of ways can avoid the profession becoming lulled into thinking that extra hours in physical education and a policy investment and commitment towards extended school day provision can be used simply for reproducing the form of provision which already exists.

SUMMARY

This is a time of change for the physical education profession. Teachers' views of what it means to be a professional are being challenged, as are aspects of their preferred beliefs and favoured teaching approaches. Therefore, the task for those with responsibility for supporting teachers with appropriate professional development opportunities is a considerable one as there is a broad and diverse range of needs at teacher, pupil and school level. Initial teacher education institutions can help in preparing teachers by providing a more differentiated curriculum and developing closer and more coherent links with schools and teacher mentors. In this way, the perceived dislocation between the academic and professional can be reduced. This chapter has also attempted to present ideas about the ways in which student teachers and more experienced teachers can develop their professional knowledge and skills. This has been attempted through identifying some of the issues most frequently associated with improving in-school and out of school collaborative learning. In addition, the challenges of developing partnership approaches with interested parties in the health and sporting communities have been reviewed, especially in relation to how physical education teachers might work effectively with other professionals at a time when pupil interest is becoming a more complex factor to include in planning programmes. In the concluding chapter, many of these ideas are further developed in order to signpost the types of future circumstance which might beckon for physical education.

CHAPTER 5

What Future for
Physical Education?

Introduction

In many respects, physical education will be continuing today in ways which are familiar to many people and which have become an established part of schooling. Classes will be grouped together in some way and 'the comforting familiarity of periods, timetables and bells' (MacBeath, 2008, p. 939) will provide the organising basis for the annual roll out of a relative familiar pattern of provision. This consistent approach to education will bring order and stability to the lives of many pupils and, of course, to the lives of many teachers as well. Within this ordered setting, many pupils will enjoy and be thoroughly engaged in well run and sympathetically delivered physical education programmes. However, as this book has tried to highlight, physical education is a complex concern, especially as it is currently close to the centre of various powerful change agendas. Thus physical education, like other subjects, will require constructing reform priorities which try to build on existing strengths during a period of curriculum renewal. So, while the 'typical' 40-year-old physical education teacher in Scotland might have experienced much in nearly two decades of teaching – the bedding in of physical education as part of Standard Grade provision, the locating of physical education as part of the 5–14 Expressive Arts, the introduction of awards at higher level and the development of new networking arrangements with the extended school community – there is a sense that physical education is on the cusp of even greater change in order to try and become a more connected component part of pupils' overall education. Thus, in the final chapter the type of future which might exist for physical education in terms of policy aspirations, teaching practices and professional development is discussed.

Future policy directions in physical education

At the outset in Chapter 1, the scale of the policy changes intended for physical education were briefly outlined with concerns highlighted about the extent to which planned changes might be subject to a degree of policy slippage as arguments continued about aims and values. Following a more detailed review of 'official' and 'unofficial' policy voices in Chapter 2, it is now worth reviewing the extent to which policy has progressed in clear and coherent ways or the extent to which policy debates are still characterised by confusion and contestation, and the implications this is likely to have for future policy directions in physical education.

At present, while the profession eagerly awaits the upsurge in provision of primary physical education which is promised, and which has been facilitated through the increased availability of professional programmes focusing on developmentally appropriate initiatives, a more familiar cycle of responsibilities is likely to be influencing secondary school teachers. This will probably involve teachers' planning for the next major curriculum reform at a time when the implementation challenges of previous curriculum changes have yet to be fully met and become part of effective practice. Thus, for example, even though there are remaining concerns about teachers' levels of content knowledge, use of appropriate methodologies and formative feedback in examination awards, it is now likely that professional development priorities will cycle forward to considering in greater detail the implementation of CfE and the new General awards which are scheduled to replace Standard Grade. In some senses 'unofficial voices', for example, teachers and academics, are insufficiently loud and organised to draw attention to those with 'official' policy making responsibilities about many of the unresolved pedagogy and professional issues which require further support.

Such is the speed of the cycle of ongoing curriculum reform that Higher Still awards have moved from being the newest to the most established part of the curriculum in a relatively short space of time. Perhaps, inevitably, this creates the impression of turbulence and a degree of ongoing confusion and disquiet rather than of fully ensuring that changes in policy do lead to changes in effective practice. Thus, there is a continuing sense of policy slippage and also a sense as well of some disappointment. For example, the aspiration that through practical experiential learning pupils could achieve greater opportunity and progression in Higher Still awards remains unfilled in many cases (Thorburn and Collins, 2006a). Ideally, the situation within examination awards would invoke a wider policy review about the appropriateness of pupils' learning experiences at a time when many pupils are preparing for the self-study demands required in higher education, but there is little evidence of this occurring at present.

Furthermore, the cycle of reform seems certain to continue unabated as the change of subject emphasis in official policy reform (e.g. CfE) encourages physical education to play a pivotal role in educating pupils to take more active responsibility for their own health and well-being. For core programmes of physical education, which have frequently been 'withering on the vine' over recent years, with a lack of curriculum guidelines in the middle years of secondary school hindering as much as helping progressions in teaching and learning, a more promising future might beckon. Therefore, a current priority is how can the policy opportunity created by a commitment towards having two hours a week of physical education become a building block for increasing levels of lifelong active learning? In addition, how will this opportunity reveal a connectivity and clarity that was largely missing from the mixed message reporting of the Review Group report (Scottish Executive, 2004a)? In pursuing such policy priorities, questions about the extent to which the subject is prepared to become integrated with health and well-being agendas will be crucial to investigate further.

In this respect, it would be helpful if curriculum developers and teachers could try to interrogate in a little greater detail what is intended by the four CfE capacities. However, achieving this is not helped by the general opaqueness of the adjectives deployed when describing pupils as 'learners', 'individuals', 'citizens' and 'contributors'. Clearly something is intended to be conveyed about the distinctiveness of the contribution each capacity offers, but the limited nature of the elaborations provided so far raises questions about how CfE will be interpreted by teachers, and to some extent understood by other key stakeholders in the policy process such as HMIE. In this environment, it is of some concern that the four capacities are set to become routine speak within physical education through the narrative privilege the 'official' policy community possesses in framing discussion (Humes, 2008), even though very few teachers might actually understand with any certainty what learning experiences might accompany the prescribed learning outcomes at this time.

Surrounded by this degree of confusion about the precise aims and conceptions of physical education being advanced, it is to be expected that many teachers might continue to reproduce programmes which reflect their own beliefs about the subject. Green (2000) has highlighted that teachers' philosophies of practice often centre on enjoyment in participation through the learning of motor skills. However, it is likely that something more than gaining a sense of release from the pressures of schooling and a reaffirmation of the physical and motor benefits of practical activity is intended to inform the enhanced curriculum inclusion of physical education. Thus, it would clearly be advantageous if the investment in primary age developmentally appropriate physical education programmes could yield substantive confirming data at key transition stages in pupils development that improved motor competence was a pivotal influence in increasing levels of active lifelong learning to a greater extent than occurs at present. Such evidence could help promote the idea that increases in secondary school curriculum time should be deployed in imaginative and new ways rather than in just doubling the time spent on the programme arrangements which already exists. Reviewed in this way, it is possible to anticipate how the pursuit of 'lifestyle activities' could merge with the continued curriculum inclusion of competitive team games (Penney and Jess, 2004).

More widely, it appears certain that the reverberations of CfE will influence practice in physical education in a number of future ways which are every bit as problematic as they are advantageous. A criticism of schools in general is that the focus on 'successful learning' has been emphasised more that the other three capacities (Hayward, 2007). For the situation to change there is a need for subjects (or curriculum areas) to design and implement learning opportunities which can authentically capture the essence of all the capacities in ways which are not stifled by contrived learning experiences or by the assessment process. Two decades ago the architects of Standard Grade physical education wanted to formally assess affective development, so crucial was it considered to be to the ways in which learning was intended to be experienced by pupils. However, the then Scottish Examination Board considered this infeasible and consequently affective development remained as a prescribed course outcome but not as a formally assessed outcome. It is doubtful, given the strength of the holistic aims ascribed to CfE, whether this would be the case today. Therefore, the opportunity exists, perhaps as never before, to assemble curricula which reflect the spirit informing CfE; where learning is active, frequently socially constructed and where experiences relate to the world beyond schools and which reflect more established notions of physical education as well. Yet, quite how such expectations can be realised when CfE is required to butt up against end-of-school examinations at higher level has yet to be adequately reviewed. Clearly, it would be helpful if teachers' inspirational teaching could triumph over anxiousness about assessment results and the negative impact this can have on the quality of teaching and learning. Some of the reported rote learning and assessment procedures experienced by pupils in higher level examinations represent a dispiriting endpoint for 15 years of school physical education (Thorburn and Collins, 2003).

However, the ways in which improvements might be managed could be influenced by the revision of Principal Teacher posts which is under way. This has frequently resulted in new faculty management arrangements with some local authorities now advertising exclusively for Principal Teacher posts in the nine identified curriculum areas of CfE rather than for single-subject Principal Teachers as previously. This arrangement, coupled with current focus on CfE, could create a situation where teachers' concerns about specific physical education matters are less likely to be directly considered than previously.

A further concern is the policy slippage associated with the 2007 manifesto commitments made by the Scottish National Party (SNP). Not only are there problems in delivering on the policy intention to provide two hours of physical education per week, there is also difficulty in providing free access to local authority swimming pools. By the beginning of 2009, only two of Scotland's thirty-two local authorities provided free year-round access. For some the nationalistic pride in securing the Commonwealth Games of 2014 might be seen as a supporting argument for legitimising Scotland as a national entity. However, for others it highlights, in plainer terms, the need for manifesto commitments in physical activity and physical education to be delivered as a foundation for achieving higher levels of sporting excellence and active life-long learning. Thus, while there is a commitment towards more outcomes-driven efficiency, as evidenced by the merging of the Scottish Institute of Sport with Sport Scotland, and a recognition that delaying full implementation of CfE would placate teachers' concerns about lack of clarity about curriculum aims and experiences, it may well be some time before some of the complex tensions which immediately impact on the practice of physical education in schools will be specifically addressed.

In the meantime, as physical education has had a curriculum presence in most forms of schooling for many years, it is easy to consider why some physical educationalists might advise caution in effectively becoming subsumed within health and well-being as part of CfE, especially given the superficial and fairly modest ways in which previous health curriculum have informed and contributed to secondary education (Forrest, 2008). However, there is a momentum of sorts behind policy intentions to 'make a difference', and this coupled with changes in how secondary schools are organised and managed looks likely to continue to exert a considerable pressure on the practice of physical education. This will invoke questions about the extent to which physical education is really committed to transformational change driven by current social justice agendas. Views will inevitably be contested on the detail of this matter. However, for those recommending caution and scepticism about the potential of physical education to contribute towards the realisation of increased equality and opportunity, it might be that through reviewing the future teaching of physical education that change agendas could be better understood and appreciated.

The future teaching of physical education

A well known feature of the policy process is that policy is easier to change than practice. Therefore, the extent to which CfE and AifL guidelines will impact on practice are still unknown. What appears to matter is whether teachers believe that the reasons for change are valid, feasible and will enhance pupils' learning experiences. In making improvements in this direction, reflecting on the broad range of learning objectives possible within physical education appears merited. This avoids too narrow a focus and on creating teaching environments where pupils are merely 'busy, happy and good' (Placek, 1983). A more fundamental debate on beliefs and values should move attention away from issues about the content in physical education and redirect attention towards teaching and learning; as research indicates that the way to improve pupils' achievement in schools is to improve teaching and learning. In short, better teachers make better schools (Teaching and Learning Research Programme, 2006).

In order to improve teaching and learning, it is not enough to simply provide teachers with alternative teaching strategies, teachers have to be provided with support so that they can be encouraged by policy makers, teacher educators and senior management staff alike to develop a culture of inquiry about their practice. This allows teachers to reflect on evidence from their own practice (and the practice of others) in developing their pedagogical knowledge. This matters as there is evidence that those teachers who adopt an inquiry approach when teaching are more able to promote active engagement in pupils' learning as well as increase pupils' autonomy and independence (Teaching and Learning Research Programme, 2006). Developing a culture of inquiry and engaging with evidence from one's own practice can also be supported, and enhanced, through collaborations with teacher educators from teacher education institutions. This approach will inform teachers about the empirical evidence which supports their practice. Developing a deeper level of understanding about practice, research and theory can be an important step in enhancing knowledge, beliefs and values about teaching. These are critical factors in improving teachers' willingness and ability to review changing the way they teach.

Ultimately, such inquiry, collaboration, research and knowledge should provide teachers with the tools needed to enable them to place the learner at the heart of the decisions they make about teaching, with decisions additionally informed by pupils' prior knowledge and experiences. By improving their understanding of the complex theories of learning highlighted in Chapter 3, for example, constructivism, teachers will begin to use their understanding of the complexities of learning alongside their knowledge of teaching and assessment practices. This may also encourage teachers to collaborate more with pupils so that they have a deeper understanding and are more alert to their individual needs and capabilities. Moreover, such improvements should reveal the importance of developing learning communities in physical education lessons, where collaborations between pupils are encouraged and where pupils develop higher cognitive understanding, improved social relations and increased self-esteem. Physical education lessons are well suited to group learning, particularly in team games as every pupil can make a contribution to the learning process. Typically, team games focus on developing individuals' ability to improve technical skills, however, by carefully selecting the teams, and by setting problems that require discussion, debate and evaluation, teachers can provide pupils with a wider range of abilities and opportunities to make a more complete contribution to the learning and the success of the team. This approach is one which is endorsed by the teaching approaches highlighted in Chapter 3, for example, TGfU (Bunker and Thorpe, 1982). Disappointingly, to date, there is little evidence that physical education teachers in Scotland adopt such approaches.

Thus, those involved in physical education, from policy makers to teachers, should be alert to the possible benefits of change. This will require a change of culture and a sharper focus on learners and learning. Change should be informed by the teacher's own practice, and through collaborations with other teachers and teacher educators. This will enhance their skills of inquiry and their understanding of empirical research and teaching and learning theory. If this happens, teachers will be better equipped to examine and develop their knowledge, beliefs and values about teaching, and ultimately, to consider bringing about changes in their teaching behaviours.

The future of professionalism in physical education

Despite the acknowledged ongoing difficulties which exist between academic and professional interpretations about what represents effective and appropriate teacher education programmes, there is evidence of more constructive and collaborative learning gains occurring when reviewing aspects of professional development for experienced teachers. For example, developmental programmes of physical education provide positive signs of the research, policy and practice communities beginning to working productively together. In this respect, progress appears better than the situation apparent for examination awards, where policy slippage is matched by lack of adequate professional development opportunities and in CfE where vagueness about possible ways of achieving learning outcomes has yet to lead to increased teacher autonomy being encouragingly grasped as part of a wider redefinition of professionalism.

However, for progress to be sustained in the longer term, continued leadership and direction will be required, for as Raffe *et al.*, (2002; 2007) discovered in their analysis of curriculum change in Scotland during the 1990s, a lack of shared vision led to a mix of political, institutional and epistemological barriers adversely affecting the levels of change expected. Therefore, the onus will be on researchers, policy makers and practitioners alike to explore continually and to review systematically the potential of curriculum experiences and pedagogical interventions in physical education to meet the changing lives and lifestyles of young people in Scotland for many years to come. If this type of critical thinking fails to occur, it will be difficult for the forces of conservatism, which are widely embedded in aspects of the teaching profession, to be overtaken.

More widely, the sense of working together to overtake challenges applies to interventions aimed at increasing participation as part of the extended school day also. A starting point in this respect is recognising that youth culture appears more complex today than in previous years. Therefore the solutions which worked in the 1980s, before a period of industrial action led to a severe reduction in teacher volunteerism, cannot be assumed to work nowadays. Developing more informed partnership approaches with professionals and volunteers in the extended school community appears necessary, as does taking more active steps to ask for, and to listen to, pupils' views more about the types of physical activity and sporting opportunities they wish.

However, while encouraging an increase in working together, continuing concerns exist about the close association and privileged access some policy entrepreneurs can have to the policy making process. This process is of potential concern as it appears to possess little in the way of the usual democratic checks expected of the normal policy process (Humes, 2008). Accordingly, in order that the practice of physical education avoids becoming unduly influenced by value-laden and agenda-driven entrepreneurial associations, it would be useful for the professional good of teachers if they could, as proactively as possible, coherently outline how government targets can be realised in ways which meet with the broad approval of physical education teachers and which promote the educational merits of pupils' learning experiences.

CONCLUSION

Achieving policy and practice gains has often been difficult due to the fragmented and often contradictory beliefs about physical education which exist. Lack of clarity and consensus about the central importance of physical education and school sport by the respective education, health and sporting communities has made it difficult, in the continuing absence of clear and sustained leadership and more robust monitoring of policy, for progress to be reflected in improved teaching and professional development opportunities. Furthermore, a lack of investment has led at times to a situation where policy makers remain pleased with the endeavours of their thinking but bemoan the delays and frustrations which often accompany policy implementation at local authority and school level. To date, less than 10% of Scottish schools have met the two hour target for physical education each week, for example (Audit Scotland, 2008). Clearly, there are tensions in deploying a policy model which is based on national programmes defining policy and setting targets coupled with locally democratic unitary authority implementation. Accordingly, it will be interesting in future years to review whether Scotland is truly committed towards the centrality of health and well-being, with quality physical education programmes as a crucial component part of this vision, or whether a narrower and perhaps more cost-effective curriculum with a bias towards examination results is preferred. This is a matter about which physical educationalists should monitor and review as part of professional practice.

The seriousness of this matter is emphasised by noting that not all countries trying to improve the triptych of 'physical education', 'physical activity' and 'youth sport' have chosen to invest so heavily in physical education. Notably, in England, matters have been viewed more widely through intentions and targets to improve activity levels throughout the entire week (in and beyond school) and through bringing staff other than physical education teachers into schools to offer practical activities. This policy idea has developed on the basis that for some pupils it is the traditions and practices of physical education itself which are the problem and, this being so, standard teaching practices are not considered the best remedy for increasing physical activity rates and youth sport participation levels. Viewed in this way, it is possible to see why physical educationalists in Scotland should be buoyed up by recognising the extent to which they have been identified for the present as a major part of the policy solution. However, this situation can change quickly, especially in the volatile political times which are likely to be ahead as the country enters a severe economic downturn. Therefore, it is important that physical education does not become 'isolated' in policy and practice terms from Scottish Governments attempts to deliver on a plethora of health, education and sporting targets, but remains central to high quality and value for money definitions of professionalism. In many respects, the opportunities of the present time have never been greater, provided, of course, that the baton for change is picked up and securely grasped.

REFERENCES

Alderman, M. K. (2003) *Motivation for Achievement: Possibilities for Teaching and Learning*. Mahwah, NJ: Lawrence Erlbaum Associates

Allison, S. and Thorpe, R. (1997) 'A comparison of the effectiveness of two approaches to teaching games within physical education: a skills approach versus a games for understanding approach', *British Journal of Physical Education*, Vol. 28, No. 3, pp. 9–13

Ames, C. (1992) 'Classroom: goals, structures and student motivation', *Journal of Educational Psychology*, Vol. 84, pp. 261–71

Anderson, R. (1999) 'The history of Scottish education, pre-1980', in Bryce and Humes (eds) (1999a), pp. 215–24

Armour, K. M. (2002) 'Stuck places: interviewing physical education teachers', paper presented at the American Education Research Association Annual Meeting, New Orleans, USA, 1–5 April

Armour, K. M. and Jones, R. L. (1998) *Physical Education Teachers' Lives and Careers*, London: Falmer Press

Armour, K. M. and Yelling, M. (2004) 'Professional "development" and professional "learning": bridging the gap for experienced physical education teachers', *European Physical Education Review*, Vol. 10, No. 1, pp. 71–93

Audit Scotland (2008) *A Performance Overview of Scottish Sport*, Edinburgh: Audit Scotland

Bailey, R., Armour, K., Kirk, D., Jess, M., Pickup, I. and Sanford, R. (2009) 'The educational benefits claimed for physical education and school sport: an academic review', *Research Papers in Education*, Vol. 24, No. 1, pp. 1–26

Ball, S. (2008) *The Education Debate: Policy and Politics in the Twenty-First Century*, Bristol: Policy Press

Bilsborough, P. and MacLeod, D. (1998) 'Standard Grade physical education: some Scottish reflections', British Journal of Physical Education, Vol. 29, No. 1, pp. 22–5

Blomqvist, M., Vanttinen, T. and Luhtanen, P. (2005) 'Assessment of secondary school students' decision-making and game play ability in soccer', *Physical Education and Sport Pedagogy*, Vol. 10, No. 2, pp. 107–19

Boyd, B. (2005) *CPD: Improving Professional Practice*, Paisley: Hodder Gibson

Boyd, B. (2008) 'The structure of the secondary curriculum', in Bryce and Humes (eds) (2008), pp. 424–34

Brewer, B. (2003) 'Physical education and sport', in Bryce and Humes (eds) (2003), pp. 588–92

Brewer, B. (2008) 'Physical education and sport', in Bryce and Humes (eds) (2008), pp. 546–50

Brewer, B. and Sharp, B. (1999b) 'Physical education', in Bryce and Humes (eds) (1999a), pp. 541–5

Bryce, T. G. K. and Humes, W. H. (eds) (1999a) *Scottish Education*, Edinburgh: Edinburgh University Press

Bryce, T.G. K. and Humes, W .H. (1999b) 'Scottish secondary education: philosophy and practice', in Bryce and Humes (eds) (1999a), pp. 37–48

Bryce, T. G. K. and Humes, W. H. (eds) (2003) *Scottish Education Second Edition: Post-Devolution*, Edinburgh: Edinburgh University Press

Bryce, T. G. K. and Humes, W. H. (eds) (2008) *Scottish Education Third Edition: Beyond Devolution*, Edinburgh: Edinburgh University Press

Bunker, D. and Thorpe, R. (1982) 'A model for the teaching of games in secondary schools', *Bulletin of Physical Education*, Vol. 18, pp. 7–10

Butler, J. I. and McCahan, B. J. (2005) 'Teaching games for understanding as a curriculum model', in Griffin, L. and Butler, J. (eds) (2005) *Teaching Games for Understanding: Theory, Research, and Practice*, Champaign, IL: Human Kinetics, pp. 33–54

Cairney, J. (2004) 'Twenty wasted years for PE in Scotland', Viewpoint, *Times Educational Supplement*, 27 August

Capel, S. (2000) 'Approaches to teaching games', in Capel, S. and Piotrowski, S. (eds) (2000) *Issues in Physical Education*, London: RoutledgeFalmer, pp. 81–98

Capel, S. (2007) 'Moving beyond physical education subject knowledge to develop knowledgeable teachers of the subject', *The Curriculum Journal*, Vol. 18, No. 4, pp. 493–507

Carpenter, P. J. and Morgan, K. (1999) 'Motivational climate, personal goal perspectives and cognitive and affective responses in physical education classes', *European Journal of Physical Education*, Vol. 4, pp. 31–41

Chow, J. Y., Davids, K., Button, C., Shuttleworth, R., Renshaw, I. and Araújo, D. (2007) 'The role of nonlinear pedagogy in physical education', *Review of Educational Research*, Vol. 77, No. 3, pp. 251–78

Coalter, F. (2007) *A Wider Role for Sport*, London: Routledge

Coalter, F., Radtke, S., Taylor, J. and Jarvie, G. (2006) *How to Achieve a Sporting Culture of Excellence in Scotland*, The Scottish Institute of Sport Foundation – a report by the Department of Sport Studies, Stirling: University of Stirling

Coalter, F. and Thorburn, M. (2003) *An Evaluation of the School Sport Co-ordinator Programme in Scotland*, Research Report No. 87, Edinburgh: Sport Scotland

Cothran, D. J., Hodges Kulinna, P., Banville, D., Choi, E., Amade-Escot, C., MacPhail, A., Macdonald, D., Richard, J-F., Sarmento, P. and Kirk, D. (2005) 'A cross-cultural investigation of the use of teaching styles', *Research Quarterly for Exercise and Sport*, Vol. 76, No. 2, pp. 193–201

Curtner-Smith, M. D. and Meek, G. A. (2000) 'Teachers' value orientations and their compatibility with the national curriculum for physical education', *European Physical Education Review*, Vol. 6, No. 1, pp. 27–45

Davids, K., Araujo, D., Button, C. and Renshaw, I. (2007) 'Degenerate brains, intermediate behaviour and representative tasks: implications for experimental design in sport psychology research', in Reilly, T., Cabri, J. and Araujo, D. (eds) (2007) *Science and Football V*, London: Routledge, pp. 537–50

Department for Culture, Media and Sport / Department for Education and Skills (2006) *The Results of the 2005/2006 School Sport Survey*, London: DCMS/DfES

Dodds, P., Griffin, L. L. and Placek, J. H. (2001) 'A selected review of the literature on development of learners' domain-specific knowledge', *Journal of Teaching in Physical Education*, Vol. 21, pp. 177–92

Donn, G. (2008) 'The political administration of Scottish education: Parliament and SEED, 2003–7', in Bryce and Humes (eds) (2008), pp. 113–22

Douglas, M. (1998) 'Comments on the marking of Higher Grade Physical Education', *Scottish Journal of Physical Education*, Vol. 26, No. 1, pp. 49–57

Dweck, C. S. and Leggett, E. L. (1988) 'A social-cognitive approach to motivation and personality', *Psychological Review*, Vol. 95, No. 2, pp. 256–73

Ennis, C. (1999) 'Creating a culturally relevant curriculum for disengaged girls', *Sport Education and Society*, Vol. 4, No. 1, pp. 31–49

Evans, J. (2004) 'Making a difference? Education and "ability" in physical education', *European Physical Education Review*, Vol. 10, No. 1, pp. 95–108

Fairclough, S. (2003) 'Physical activity, perceived competence and enjoyment during high school physical education', *European Journal of Physical Education*, Vol. 8, pp. 5–18

Fairclough, S. and Stratton, S. (2005) 'Physical activity levels in middle and high school physical education: a review', *Pediatric Exercise Science*, Vol. 17, pp. 217–36

Forrest, J. (2008) 'Health promotion', in Bryce and Humes (eds) (2008), pp. 490–5

Gallahue, D. (1982) *Developmental Movement Experiences for Children*, New York: Wiley

Gard, M. (2004) 'An elephant in the room and a bridge too far, or physical education and the "obesity epidemic"', in Evans, J., Davies, B. and Burrows, L. (eds) (2004), *Body Knowledge and Control: Studies in the Sociology of Physical Education and Health*, London: Routledge, pp. 68–82

Gower, C. and Capel, S. (2004) 'Newly qualified physical education teachers' experiences of developing subject knowledge prior to, during and after a Postgraduate Certificate in Education course', *Physical Education and Sport Pedagogy*, Vol. 9, No. 2, pp. 165–83

Graham, G., Holt-Hale, S. and Parker, M. (1980) *Children Moving*, Mountain View, CA: Mayfield Press

Gray, S. (2008) 'Team invasion games within the Scottish physical education curriculum: rhetoric, reality and implications for policy', unpublished doctoral thesis: University of Edinburgh

Gray, S., Sproule, J. and Wang, J. C. K. (2008) 'Pupils' perceptions of and experiences in team invasion games: a case study of a Scottish secondary school and its three feeder primary schools', *European Physical Education Review*, Vol. 14, No. 2, pp. 179–201

Green, K. (1998) 'Philosophies, ideologies and the practice of physical education', *Sport, Education and Society*, Vol. 3 No. 2, pp. 125–43

Green, K. (2000) 'Exploring the everyday "philosophies" of physical education teachers from a sociological perspective', *Sport, Education and Society*, Vol. 5, No. 2, pp. 109–29

Green, K. (2002a) 'Physical education and the couch potato society', *European Journal of Physical Education*, Vol. 7, No. 2, pp. 95–107

Green, K. (2002b) 'Lifelong participation, physical education and the work of Ken Roberts', *Sport, Education and Society*, Vol. 7, No. 2, pp. 167–82

Green, K. (2008) *Understanding Physical Education*, London: Sage

Green, K. and Lamb, K. (2000) 'Health-related exercise, effort perception and physical education', *European Journal of Physical Education*, Vol. 5, No. 1, pp. 88–103

Griffin, L. L., Mitchell, S. A. and Oslin, J. L. (1997) *Teaching Sport Concepts and Skills*, Champaign, IL: Human Kinetics

Griffin, L. M. and Combs, S. C. (2000) 'Student teachers' perceptions of the role of the physical educator', *Journal of Physical Education, Recreation & Dance*, Vol. 71, pp. 42–5

Hardman, K. and Marshall, J. J. (2000) *World-wide Survey of the State and Status of School*

Physical Education, Final Report, Manchester: University of Manchester

Hardman, K. and Marshall, J. J. (2005) 'Physical education in schools in European context', in Green, K. and Hardman, K. (eds) (2005), *Physical Education: Essential Issues*, London: Sage, pp. 39–64

Hastie, P. A. (1996) 'Student role involvement during a unit of sport education', *Journal of Teaching in Physical Education*, Vol. 16, No. 1, pp. 88–103

Hastie, P. A. (1998) 'The participation and perception of girls within a unit of sport education', *Journal of Teaching in Physical Education*, Vol. 17, pp. 157–71

Hastie, P. A. (2004) 'Problem-solving in teaching sports', in Wright, J., Macdonald, D. and Burrows, L. (eds) (2004)*Critical Inquiry and Problem-Solving in Physical Education*, London: Routledge, pp. 62–73

Hayward, L. and Hedge, N. (2005) 'Travelling towards change in assessment: policy, practice and research in education', *Assessment in Education*, Vol. 12, No. 1, pp. 55–75

Hayward, L. (2007) 'Curriculum, pedagogies and assessment in Scotland: the quest for social justice "Ah kent yir faither"', *Assessment in Education*, Vol. 14, No. 2, pp. 251–68

Hepburn, H. (2009) 'A case of all talk and no action', *Times Educational Supplement (Scotland)*, 16 January

Her Majesty's Inspectorate of Education (2001) *Improving Physical Education in Primary Schools*, Edinburgh: HMSO

Her Majesty's Inspectorate of Education (2008) *Physical Education: A portrait of current practice in Scottish schools and pre-school centres* (online). Available at URL: http://www.hmie.gov.uk/documents/publication/pepcp.html (accessed 12 January 2009)

Holt, N. L., Strean, W. B. and Bengoechea, E. G. (2002) 'Expanding the teaching games for understanding model: new avenues for future research and practice', *Journal of Teaching in Physical Education*, Vol. 21, pp. 162–76

Hopper, T. (2002) 'Teaching games for understanding: The importance of student emphasis over content emphasis', *Journal of Physical Education, Recreation and Dance*, Vol. 73, No. 7, pp. 44–8

Houlihan, B. and Green, M. (2006) 'The changing status of school sport and physical education: explaining policy change', *Sport, Education and Society*, Vol. 11, No. 1, pp. 73–92

Humes, W. (1999) 'Policy making in Scottish education', in Bryce and Humes (eds) (1999a), pp. 73–82

Humes, W. (2003) 'Policy making in Scottish education', in Bryce and Humes (eds) (2003), pp. 74–85

Humes, W. (2008) 'Policy making in Scottish education', in Bryce and Humes (eds) (2008), pp. 69–79

Humes, W. and Bryce, T. (1999) 'The distinctiveness of Scottish education', in Bryce and Humes (eds) (1999a), pp. 102–11

Jess, M. (2004) 'The future of physical education in Scotland: the report of the National Review Group', *British Journal of Teaching Physical Education*, Vol. 35, No. 2, pp. 6–9

Jess. M. and Collins, D. (2003) 'Primary physical education in Scotland: the future in the making', *European Journal of Physical Education*, Vol. 8, No. 1, pp. 103–18

Johns, D. (2005) 'Recontextualizing and delivering the biomedical model as a physical education curriculum', *Sport Education and Society*, Vol. 10, No. 1, pp. 69–84

Jones, C. and Farrow, D. (1999) 'The transfer of strategic knowledge: a test of the games classification curriculum model', *Bulletin of Physical Education*, Vol. 35, No. 2, pp. 103–24

Kennedy, A. (2008) 'The professional development of teachers', in Bryce and Humes eds) (2008), p. 836–46

Kirk, D. (1988) *Physical Education and Curriculum Study: A Critical Introduction*, London: Croom Helm

Kirk, D. (2002) 'Physical education: a gendered history', in Penney, D. (ed.) (2002) *Gender and Physical Education: Contemporary Issues and Future Directions*, London: Routledge, pp. 24–37

Kirk, D. (2004) 'New practices, new subjects and critical inquiry', in Wright, J., MacDonald, D. and Burrows, L. (eds) (2004) *Critical Inquiry and Problem Solving in Physical Education*, London: Routledge, pp. 199–208

Kirk, D. (2005) 'Future prospects for teaching games for understanding', in Griffin, L. and Butler, J. (eds) (2005) *Teaching Games for Understanding: Theory, Research, and Practice*, Champaign, IL: Human Kinetics, pp. 213–27

Kirk, D. (2006) 'The "obesity crises" and school physical education', *Sport Education and Society*, Vol. 11 No. 2, pp. 121–33

Kirk, D. and MacPhail, A. (2002) 'Teaching games for understanding and situated learning: re-thinking the Bunker-Thorpe model', *Journal of Teaching in Physical Education*, Vol. 21, No. 4, pp. 177–92

Klint, K. A. and Weiss, M. R. (1987) 'Perceived competence and motives for participating in youth sports: A test of Harter's competence motivation theory', *Journal of Sport Psychology*, Vol. 9, pp. 55–65

Kretchmar, S. R. (2000) 'Moving and being moved: implications for practice', *Quest*, Vol. 43, No. 2, pp. 78–97

Kulinna, P. H. and Cothran, D. J. (2003) 'Physical education teachers' self-reported use and perceptions of various teaching styles', *Learning and Instruction*, Vol. 13, pp. 597–609

Laker, A. (2000) *Beyond the Boundaries of Physical Education: Educating Young People for Citizenship and Social Responsibility*, London: Routledge

Lawson, H. A. (1986) 'Occupational socialisation and the design of teacher education programs', *Journal of Teaching in Physical Education*, Vol. 5, No. 2, pp. 107–16

Lee, M. (2004) 'Values in physical education and sport: a conflict of interests?', *British Journal of Teaching Physical Education*, Vol. 35, No. 1, pp. 6–10

Lewin, B. (2005) *Reforming Education: From Origins to Outcomes*, London: RoutledgeFalmer

Li, W., Lee, A. and Solmon, M. (2007) 'The role of perceptions of task difficulty in relation to self-perceptions of ability, intrinsic value, attainment value, and performance', *European Physical Education Review*, Vol. 13, No. 3, pp. 301–18

Light, R. (2008) 'Complex learning theory – its epistemology and its assumptions about learning: implications for physical education', *Journal of Teaching in Physical Education*, Vol. 27, pp. 21–37

Light, R. and Fawns, R. (2001) 'The thinking body: constructivist approaches to games teaching in physical education', *Melbourne Studies in Education*, Vol. 42, No. 2, pp. 69–97

Light, R. and Wallian, N. (2008) 'A constructivist-informed approach to teaching swimming', *Quest*, Vol. 60, No. 3, pp. 387–404

Littlefield, R., Green, B., Forsyth, S. and Sharp, B. (2003) 'Physical education in Scottish schools – a national case study', *European Journal of Physical Education*, Vol. 8, pp. 211–27

Livingston, K. and Robertson, J. (2001) 'The coherent system and the empowered individual: continuing professional development for teachers in Scotland', *European Journal of Teacher Education*, Vol. 24, pp. 183–94

McCrone, D. (2003) 'Culture, nationalism and Scottish education: homogeneity and diversity', in Bryce and Humes (eds) (2003), pp. 239–49

MacBeath, J. (2008) 'Do schools have a future?', in Bryce and Humes (eds) (2008), pp. 939–48

MacDonald, S. (2008) 'The tycoon is handing out his treatise on success to every Scottish pupil' (online). Available at URL: www.timesonline.co.uk/tol/news/uk/scotland/article4692350.ece (accessed 20 December 2008)

MacLean, J. (2007) 'A longitudinal study to ascertain the factors that impact on the confidence of undergraduate physical education student teachers to teach dance in Scottish schools', *European Physical Education Review*, Vol. 13, No. 1, pp. 99–116

MacPhail, A. (2004) The social construction of Higher Grade Physical Education: the impact of teacher curriculum decision-making, *Sport Education and Society*, Vol. 9, No. 1, pp. 55–73

MacPhail, A. (2007) 'Teachers' views on the construction, management and delivery of an externally prescribed physical education curriculum: Higher Grade Physical Education', *Physical Education and Sport Pedagogy*, Vol. 12, No. 1, pp. 43–60

McMahon, E. and MacPhail, A. (2007) 'Learning to teach sport education: the experience of a pre-service teacher', *European Physical Education Review*, Vol. 13, No. 2, pp. 229–46

Menter, I. (2008) 'Teacher education institutions', in Bryce and Humes (eds) (2008), pp. 817–25

Menter, I., Mahoney, P. and Hextall, I. (2004) 'Never the twain shall meet? Modernising the teaching profession in Scotland and England', *Journal of Education Policy*, Vol. 19, No. 2, pp. 196–214

Menzies, J. (1997) 'A case study of differences in attainment between boys and girls in Standard Grade Physical Education (Part 1)', *Scottish Journal of Physical Education*, Vol. 25, No. 3, pp. 34–40

Menzies, J. (1998) 'A case study of differences in attainment between boys and girls in Standard Grade Physical Education (Part 2)', *Scottish Journal of Physical Education*, Vol. 26, No. 1, pp. 29–48

Mitchell, S. A. and Oslin, J. L. (1999) 'An investigation of tactical transfer in net games', *European Journal of Physical Education*, Vol. 4, pp. 162–72

Morgan, K., Kingston, K. and Sproule, J. (2005) 'The effects of different teaching styles on the teacher behaviours that influence motivational climate in physical education', *European Physical Education Review*, Vol. 11, No. 3, pp. 257–86

Morrison, K. (2008) 'Educational philosophy and the challenge of complexity theory', *Education Philosophy and Theory*, Vol. 40, No. 1, pp. 19–34

Mosston, M. and Ashworth, S. (2002) *Teaching Physical Education* (5th edn), San Francisco, CA: Pearson Education

Munro, N. (2006) 'A healthy change of course', *Times Educational Supplement (Scotland)*, 3 November

Murdoch, E. B. (1990) 'Physical education and sport: the interface', in Armstrong, N. (ed.) (1990) *New Directions in Physical Education*, London: Cassell, pp. 63–77

Nutt, G. and Clarke, G. (2002) 'The hidden curriculum and the changing nature of teachers' work', in Laker, A. (ed.) (2002) *The Sociology of Sport and Physical Education: An Introductory Reader*, London: RoutledgeFalmer, pp. 148–66

Oslin, J. and Mitchell, S. (2006) 'Game-centred approaches to teaching physical education', in Kirk, D., Macdonald, D. and O'Sullivan, M. (eds) (2006) *The Handbook of Physical Education*, London: Sage, pp. 627–51

Ozga, J. (2005) 'Modernizing the education workforce: a perspective from Scotland', *Educational Review*, Vol. 57, No. 2, pp. 207–19

Parish L. E. and Treasure, D. (2003) 'Physical activity and situational motivation in physical education: Influence of the motivational climate and perceived ability', *Research Quarterly for Exercise and Sport*, Vol. 74, No. 2, pp. 173–82

Peacock, P. (2004) Record of Scottish Parliamentary debate on 'Educational Reform', 22 January (online). Available at URL: www.scottish.parliament.uk/business/officialreports/meetingsparliament/or- 04/sor0122- 02.htm (accessed 10 January 2009)

Penney, D. (2008) 'Playing a political game and playing for position: policy and curriculum development in health and physical education', *European Physical Education Review*, Vol. 14, No. 1, pp. 33–49

Penney. D. and Chandler, T. (2000) 'Physical education: what future(s)?', *Sport, Education and Society*, Vol. 5, No. 1, pp. 71–87

Penney, D. and Jess, M. (2004) 'Physical education and physically active lives: a lifelong approach to curriculum development', *Sport, Education and Society*, Vol. 9, No. 4, pp. 269–87

Penney, D., Jess, M. and Thorburn, M. (2006) 'Improving the house of cards: productive pressures for curriculum reform in secondary physical education', paper presented at the Australian Association for Research in Education conference, 27–30 November, Adelaide

Placek, J. H. (1983) 'Conceptions of success in teaching: busy, happy, and good?', in Templin, T. and Olsen, J. (eds) (1983) *Teaching in Physical Education*, Champaign, IL: Human Kinetics, pp. 46–56

Purdon, A. (2003) 'A national framework of CPD: continuing professional development or continuing policy dominance?', *Journal of Education Policy*, Vol. 18, No. 4, pp. 423–37

Raffe, D., Howieson, C. and Tinklin, T. (2002) 'The Scottish educational crisis of 2000: an analysis of the policy process of unification', *Journal of Education Policy*, Vol. 17, No. 2, pp. 167–85

Raffe, D., Howieson, C. and Tinklin, T. (2007) 'The impact of a unified curriculum and qualifications system: the Higher Still reform of post-16 education in Scotland', *British Educational Research Journal*, Vol. 33, No. 4, pp. 479–508

Reid, A. (1996a) 'The concept of physical education in current curriculum and assessment policy in Scotland', *European Physical Education Review*, Vol. 2, No. 1, pp. 7–18

Reid, A. (1996b) 'Knowledge, practice and theory in physical education', *European Physical Education Review*, Vol. 2, No. 2, pp. 94–104

Reid, A. (1997) 'Value pluralism and physical education', *European Physical Education Review*, Vol. 3, No. 1, pp. 6–20

Rovegno, I., Nevett, M. and Babiarz, M. (2001) 'Learning and teaching invasion game tactics in 4th grade: introduction and theoretical perspective', *Journal of Teaching in Physical Education*, Vol. 20, pp. 299–300

Sachs, J. (2003) *The Activist Teaching Profession*, Milton Keynes: Open University Press

Scottish Executive (1998) *Scottish Health Survey*, Edinburgh: Scottish Executive

Scottish Executive (2001) *A Teaching Profession for the Twenty-First Century: Report of the Committee of Inquiry into Professional Conditions of Service for Teachers* (The McCrone Report), Edinburgh: Scottish Executive

Scottish Executive (2003a) *Let's Make Scotland More Active: A Strategy for Physical Activity*. Edinburgh: Scottish Executive

Scottish Executive (2003b) *Scottish Health Survey*, Edinburgh: Scottish Executive

Scottish Executive (2003c) *Active Schools Programme*. Edinburgh: Scottish Executive

Scottish Executive (2004a) *The Report of the Review Group on Physical Education*, Edinburgh: Scottish Executive

Scottish Executive (2004b) *A Curriculum for Excellence*, Edinburgh: Scottish Executive

Scottish Executive (2004c) *Response from Peter Peacock, Minister for Education and Young People, June 15th, 2004* (online). Available at URL: www.scotland.gov.uk/Publications/2004/06/19482/38627 (accessed 11 January 2009)

Scottish Executive (2005) *Statistical Bulletin Education Series*, Edinburgh: Scottish Executive

Scottish Executive (2007) *Reaching Higher: Building on the success of Sport 2*, Edinburgh: Scottish Executive

Scottish Government (2008) *Statistical Bulletin Education Series: Teachers in Scotland 2007* (online). Available at URL: www.scotland.gov.uk/Resource/Doc/91982/0058105. pdf (accessed 14 March 2009)

Scottish Office Education Department (1992) *Expressive Arts Curriculum and Assessment in Scotland: National Guidelines*, Edinburgh: SOED

Scottish Office Education Department / HM Inspectorate of Education (1995) *Effective Learning and Teaching in Scottish Secondary Schools – Physical Education*, Edinburgh: HMSO

Sharp, R. (1990) *Physical Education in Scottish Secondary Schools: Report of a Nationwide Survey*, Glasgow: Jordanhill College

Shulman, L. S. (1987) 'Knowledge and teaching: foundations of the new reform', *Harvard Educational Review*, Vol. 57, pp. 1–22

Sicilia-Camacho, A. and Brown, D. (2008) 'Revisiting the paradigm shift from the versus to the non-versus notion of Mosston's spectrum of teaching styles in physical education pedagogy: a critical pedagogical perspective', *Physical Education and Sport Pedagogy*, Vol. 13, No. 1, pp. 85–108

Siedentop, D. (1994) 'Introduction to sport education', in Siedentop, D. (ed.) (1994) *Sport Education: Quality Physical Education through Positive Sport Experiences*, Champaign, IL: Human Kinetics, pp. 3–16

Siedentop, D. (1996) 'Physical education and education reform: The case of sport education', in Silverman S. J. and Ennis, C. D. (eds) (1996) *Student Learning in Physical Education, Applying Research to Enhance Instruction*, Champaign, IL: Human Kinetics, pp. 247–68

Siedentop, D. (2002) 'Content knowledge for physical education', *Journal of Teaching in Physical Education*, Vol. 21, No. 4, pp. 368–78

Sport Scotland (2003) *Sport 21 2003–2007: The National Strategy for Sport – Shaping Scotland's Future*, Edinburgh: Sport Scotland

Sport Scotland (2008a) *Moving Forward Together: Annual Review 2007/2008*, Edinburgh: Sport Scotland

Sport Scotland (2008b) *Fit for Girls: Case Studies*, Edinburgh: Sport Scotland

Standage, M., Treasure, D. C., Hooper, K. and Kuczka, K. (2007) 'Self-handicapping in school physical education: the influence of the motivational climate', *British Journal of Educational Psychology*, Vol. 77, No. 1, pp. 81–99

Stroot, S. A. (1996) 'Organisational socialisation: factors impacting beginning teachers', in Silverman, S. J. and Ennis, C. D. (eds) (1996) *Student Learning in Physical Education: Applying Research to Enhance Instruction*, Champaign, IL: Human Kinetics, pp. 339–66

Sutherland, Sir Stewart (1997) Report 10 – Teacher Education and Training: A Study (The Sutherland Report) in National Committee of Inquiry in Higher Education, *Higher Education in the Learning Society*, Report of the National Committee, Norwich: HMSO

Teaching and Learning Research Programme (2006) *Improving Teaching and Learning in Schools*, London: TLRP

Thelen, E. and Smith, L. B. (1994) *A Dynamic Systems Approach to the Development of Cognition and Action*, Cambridge, MA: MIT Press

Theodoulides, A. and Armour, K.A. (2001) 'Personal, social and moral development through team games: some critical questions', *European Physical Education Review*, Vol. 7, No. 1, pp. 5–23

Thomson, I. (1993) 'Physical education in Scotland, 1973–1993', *Scottish Journal of Physical Education*, Vol. 21, No. 2, pp. 4–14

Thomson, I. (1996) 'Official views on physical education and sport', *Scottish Journal of Physical Education*, Vol. 24, No. 1, pp. 41–3

Thorburn, M. (2004) 'Providing "Opportunity for All" through Higher Still: a continuing challenge for physical education in Scotland', *Scottish Educational Review*, Vol. 24, No. 1, pp. 66–78

Thorburn, M. (2005) 'Emerging models of professionalism: the changing expectations of physical education teachers in school and community settings', *Education in the North*, Vol. 13, pp. 47–53

Thorburn, M. (2006) 'The loneliness of the long distance Scottish physical education teacher: how to provide effective in-service for experienced teachers implementing new curricula', *Journal of In-service Education*, Vol. 32, No. 3, pp. 359–73

Thorburn, M. (2007a) 'Achieving conceptual and curriculum coherence in high-stakes school examinations in physical education', *Physical Education and Sport Pedagogy*, Vol. 12, No. 2, pp. 163–84

Thorburn, M. (2007b) 'Seizing the moment: improving curriculum and pedagogy prospects for physical education in Scotland', *Forum*, Vol. 49, No. 3, pp. 305–10

Thorburn, M. (2008) 'Articulating a Merleau-Pontian phenomenology of physical education: the quest for active student engagement and authentic assessment in high-stakes examination awards', Vol. 14, No. 2, pp. 263–80

Thorburn, M. (2009) 'Physical education, the policy entrepreneur and comprehensive schooling: can they exist in harmony?', *Forum* Vol. 51, No. 1, pp. 101–5

Thorburn, M. and Collins, D. (2003) 'The effects of an integrated curriculum model on teachers' pedagogy practices', *European Physical Education Review*, Vol. 9, No. 2, pp. 187–211

Thorburn, M. and Collins, D. (2006a) 'Integrated curriculum model and their effects on student learning and attainment', *European Physical Education Review*, Vol. 12, No. 1, pp. 31–50

Thorburn, M. and Collins, D. (2006b) 'Accuracy and authenticity of oral and written assessments in high-stakes school examinations', *Curriculum Journal*, Vol. 17, No. 1, pp. 3–25

Tsangaridou, N. (2008) 'Trainee primary teachers' beliefs and practices about physical education during student teaching', *Physical Education and Sport Pedagogy*, Vol. 13, No. 2, pp. 131–52

Turner, A. P. and Martinek, T. J. (1999) 'An investigation into teaching games for understanding: effect on skill, knowledge, and game play', *Research Quarterly for Exercise and Sport*, No. 70, pp. 286–96

Van Driel, J. H., Verloop, N. I. and de Vos, W. (1998) 'Developing science teachers' pedagogical content knowledge', *Journal of Research in Science Teaching*, Vol. 35, No. 6, pp. 673–95

Varela, F. J., Thompson, E. and Rosch, E. (1991), *The Embodied Mind: Cognitive Science and Human Experience*, Cambridge, MA: MIT Press

Wallhead, T. L. and Buckworth, J. (2004) 'The role of physical education in the promotion of youth physical activity', *Quest*, Vol. 56, No. 3, pp. 285–301

Weiss, M. R. and Ferrer-Caja, E. (2000) 'Predictors of intrinsic motivation amongst adolescent students in physical education', *Research Quarterly for Exercise and Sport*, Vol. 71, No. 3, pp. 267–79

Welk, G. J. (1999) 'The youth physical activity promotion model: a conceptual bridge between theory and practice', *Quest*, Vol. 51, No. 1, pp. 5–23

Whitty, G. (2006) 'Education(al) research and education policy making: is conflict inevitable?', *British Educational Research Journal*, Vol. 32, No. 2, pp. 159–76

Wigfield, A. and Eccles, J. S. (2000) 'Expectancy–value theory of achievement motivation', *Contemporary Educational Psychology*, Vol. 25, No. 1, pp. 68–81

Williams, A. M. and Hodges, N. J. (2005) 'Practice, instruction and skill acquisition: challenging tradition', *Journal of Sports Sciences*, Vol. 23, No. 6, pp. 637–50

Wright, S., McNeill, M., Fry, J. and Wang, J. (2005) 'Teaching teachers to play and teach games', *Physical Education and Sport Pedagogy*, Vol. 10, No. 1, pp. 6–82

Xiang, P., Lee, A. and Williamson, L. (2001) 'Conceptions of ability in physical education: children and adolescents', *Journal of Teaching in Physical Education*, Vol. 20, No. 2, pp. 282–94

INDEX

ability 33, 36
Active Schools Coordinators 24
Active Schools programme 24, 63, 64
activity-driven teaching 53
AifL (Assessment is for Learning) 57, 60, 73
Alderman, M. K. 33
Allison, S. 45
Ames, C. 35
Anderson, R. 8
Armour, K. M. 32, 40, 59, 60, 62
Ashworth, S. 37–8
Assessment is for Learning: see AifL
assessment process 13, 61, 71–2

Bailey, R. 46
Ball, S. 2
Basic Moves programme 23–4, 28, 34, 42
Berlin World Summit on Physical
  Education 21
Bilsborough, P. 10, 11
Blomqisvt, M. 45
Boyd, B. 49, 61
breadth vs. depth 32, 34, 36, 52–3
Brewer, B. 8, 11, 13, 15, 40, 60, 62, 63–4
Brown, D. 35
Bryce, T. G. K. 17
Buckworth, J. 27
Bunker, D. 4, 44, 74
Butler, J. I. 46

Cairney, J. 16
Capel, S. 4, 36, 39, 46, 47, 53, 54
career development 25, 56
Carpenter, P. J. 36
cascade mode of delivery 56, 57
CfE (Curriculum for Excellence) 58–9;
  constructivism 43; curriculum reforms
  17, 69; and exams 15, 28; health and
  well-being 31–2, 59; holistic aims 71;
  implementation 47, 72, 73; learning
  outcomes 46; physical education 9,
  30, 31–2; professional development 59;
  student teachers 52; teachers' remit 63
Chandler, T. 35

Chartered Teacher programme 56
Chow, J. Y. 41, 42
Clarke, G. 52
Coalter, F. 3, 25, 27, 62, 64, 65, 66
cognitive skills 33–4, 45
collaboration 51, 58, 74
collaborative working 57
Collins, D. 13, 14, 23, 24, 37, 60, 69, 72
Combs, S. C. 38
Commonwealth Games, Glasgow 22, 72
competence, actual/perceived 32, 33–4,
  35, 46
comprehensive schools 27
conditions of service 63
constraints theory 42
constructivism: CfE 43; learning
  autonomy 74; learning environment 4,
  41; movement patterns 23; swimming
  example 43; university courses 55
content knowledge 10, 11–12, 13, 40, 60
Continuing Professional Development
  (CPD) courses 39–40
Cothran, D. J. 38
critical engagement 32, 53, 75
curriculum development 62, 75
Curriculum for Excellence: see CfE
curriculum reform 17, 19–21, 69–71
curriculum resources 59
Curtner-Smith, M. D. 51

dance 54
Davids, K. 42
DCMS/DfES 53
Department of Health and Communities
  27
development officers 10, 12
developmental programmes 23–4
differentiated programmes 35–6, 54, 55
discussion 32, 43, 60
Dodds, P. 45
Donn, G. 63
Douglas, M. 10
Dunfermline College of Physical Education
  50

Dunning Report 6, 8
Dweck, C. S. 35

Eccles, J. S. 47
Edinburgh University 23, 28–9, 50, 53, 57
Education Bill (2000) 56
England, physical education 52, 76
enjoyment 34, 44, 45, 63
Ennis, C. 44
Evans, J. 53
examinations 28, 60–1;see also Higher;
 Higher Still; Standard Grade
experiential learning 14–15, 22, 53, 60, 61
Expressive Arts 5--14 16, 23
extended school days 62, 63

facilitating role 43–4, 45, 55
Fairclough, S. 19, 35
Farrow, D. 45
Fawns, R. 43
feedback 13, 14, 33, 37, 61
Ferrer-Caja, E. 33, 35
Fit for Girls (FfG) 25–6
5--14 national guidelines 16, 23, 68
Forrest, J. 72
Further Education lecturers 12

Gallahue, D. 23
game-based approaches 44, 46;see also team
 games
Gard, M. 21
gender differences 12, 25–6, 33–4, 44
General Teaching Council for Scotland: see
 GTCS
girls 12, 25–6, 33–4, 44
Girls in Sport and Physical Activity Project
 25
Gower, C. 54
graduate degree programmes 6
Graham, G. 23
Gray, S. 32, 36
Green, K. 19–20, 23, 29, 39, 52, 66, 69
Green, M. 3
Griffin, L. L. 4, 44
Griffin, L. M. 38
GTCS (General Teaching Council for
 Scotland) 27, 51, 56

Hardman, K. 16, 21
Hastie, P. A. 44
Hayward, L. 14, 61, 71
health and well-being 46; CfE 31–2, 59;
 curriculum development 62; physical

education 7, 17–28, 23, 24; responsibility
 69
health of nation 30, 77
Health Promoting Schools 63
Hedge, N. 14, 61
Hepburn, H. 5, 51, 52, 65
Her Majesty's Inspectorate of Education:
 see HMIE
Heriot-Watt University 50
Higher examinations 9–10
Higher Still 10, 11–12, 13, 15, 40, 69
Higher Still Physical Education: see HSPE
HMIE (Her Majesty's Inspectorate of
 Education) 15, 27; and CfE 19, 70;
 collaborative learning 3; policy 2;
 postgraduate programmes 51; primary
 physical education 16; professional
 development 49; seconded teachers
 10; Successful Learners 35; technique
 development 11, 37
Hodges, N. J. 37
Holt, N. L. 32
Hopper, T. 44–5
Houlihan, B. 3
HSPE (Higher Still Physical Education) 37,
 40, 60
Humes, W. H. 2, 10, 17, 69, 76

inclusive model 66
Independent schools 19
industrial action 75
initial teacher education: see ITE
intentions, embodied 41–2
ITE (initial teacher education) 39, 46, 50–5,
 61, 67

Jess, M. 19, 21, 23, 24, 53, 71
Johns, D. 21
Jones, C. 45
Jones, R. L. 62
Jordanhill College 50

Kennedy, A. 57, 59
Kirk, D. 1, 4, 11, 21, 41, 46, 53
Klint, K. A. 33
Kretchmar, S. R. 22
Kulinna, P. H. 38

Lamb, K. 23
Lawson, H. A. 38
leadership 75, 76
learning: autonomy 3, 35, 43, 58; cognitive/
 physical 31–2; context 45; needs/

approaches 35; non-linear 58; off-the-ball 45; practical 21; self-directed 35; successful 71; superficial 59; transfer 34;*see also* constructivism; experiential learning; situated learning
Learning and Teaching Scotland: *see* LTS
learning environment 41, 42–3
learning to move/moving to learn 19–20, 30
lecturers in teacher education 54
Lee, M. 22
Leggett, E. L. 35
Lewin, B. 25
Li, W. 47
lifelong learning 17, 19, 24, 30, 53, 54, 71
lifelong physical activity 5–6, 24, 30, 32
Light, R. 41, 42, 43, 47, 58
Littlefield, R. 15, 19, 32
Livingston, K. 56
Loughborough Partnership 64
LTS (Learning and Teaching Scotland) 2, 27, 29, 59

MacBeath, J. 68
McCahan, B. J. 46
McConnell, J. 26
McCrone Report 27, 54
MacDonald, S. 27
MacLean, J. 54
MacLeod, D. 10, 11
McMahon, E. 39
MacPhail, A. 4, 10, 12, 13, 39, 40, 41
Marshall, J. J. 16, 21
Martin, L. 25
Martinek, T. J. 45
Meek, G. A. 51
Menter, I. 27, 52
Menzies, J. 12
Mitchell, S. 4, 41, 45
modelling, as teaching strategy 33
Moray House School of Education 50
Morgan, K. 36
Morrison, K. 57
Mosston, M. 37–8
motivational climate 14, 33, 35–6
motor skills: context 32, 37; perceptual 11; teaching of 38, 46, 70; team games 36, 41, 44–5
movement patterns 23, 34
Munn Report 6, 8, 15
Munro, N. 17, 18
Murdoch, E. B. 66

National Curriculum of England & Wales 23
National Strategy for Sport (Scottish Executive) 22, 24
Nutt, G. 52

obesity, increasing 18, 21
Occupational Socialisation Theory 38
Oslin, J. 4, 41, 45
Ozga, J. 25

Paisley University 50
Parish, L. E. 36
participation-based approach 62, 63, 66
Peacock, P. 63
pedagogical approaches 3–6, 13, 19, 30–1, 39
Penney, D. 17, 19, 21, 24, 35, 53, 71
performance 11–12; evaluation 33; feedback 13, 14; focus on 28; knowledge and understanding 9–10; learning environment 41; practical/analytical 12–15
physical activity 20–1, 24–8; decline in 18; girls 25–6; lifelong 24, 30; national strategy 63; participation levels 66; Standard Grade 10
physical education 20–1; aims and objectives 1, 3, 8, 47; CfE 9, 30, 31–2; in curriculum 1, 15–18, 21, 31–2, 47; England 52, 76; future teaching of 73–4; health and well-being 7, 17–28, 23, 24; policy directions 68–73; status 2–3, 22; timetabled 9, 15–16, 76
physical education teachers: beliefs and attitudes 1, 4–5, 14, 38–40, 49, 69; delivering curriculum 3–4; entry candidates 52; feedback 13; health messages 23; implementation of policy 14; pedagogical approaches 13, 19, 30–1; professional development programmes 56–61; professionalism 26, 28; service agreements 6; sports-based participation 24; statistics 48–9; unionized 25
Placek, J. H. 73
placement schools 51, 53
policy 2–3, 8–9, 25–6, 29, 68–73
postgraduate study 29, 51
practical activities, range on offer 53
primary physical education 16, 29, 49, 57–8, 69, 71
Principal Teacher posts 72
problem solving 32, 36, 44

process-driven environment 42
professional development programmes 10, 20, 39, 49, 56–61
professionalism 5–6, 26, 28, 47; defined 51–2; future 75–6; improved 49
pupil-centred curriculum model 43, 66
pupil-centred learning 4, 35–6, 42–4
Purdon, A. 56

Raffe, D. 75
recruitment of new teachers 63
reflecting 32, 43
Reid, A. 11, 15
research-informed teaching 57
responsibility 43, 44, 45, 69
retirement rate 63
Review Group on Physical Education (Scottish Executive) 18, 19–20, 22–4, 31–2, 57, 65, 69
Robertson, J. 56
rote learning 13, 14, 37, 71
Rovegno, I. 45

Sachs, J. 54
school clubs 66
School Sport Coordinator Programme: see SSCP
school types 13–14
Schools Minister 20–1
Scottish Examination Board 71
Scottish Executive 16, 17, 33, 35, 48, 53, 63; Active Schools programme 24, 63; Health Promoting Schools 63; McCrone Report 54; National Strategy for Sport 22, 24; Review Group on Physical Education 18, 22–4, 31–2, 57, 65, 69; Scottish Health Survey 18
Scottish Executive Health and Education Ministers 17
Scottish Government 27, 30, 48–9, 56, 77
Scottish Health Survey (Scottish Executive) 18
Scottish Institute of Sport Foundation 27, 72
Scottish Journal of Physical Education 10
Scottish Local Authority Network of Physical Education 51
Scottish Nationalist Party manifesto 22, 72
Scottish Parliament 17, 27
Scottish Qualifications Authority: see SQA
Scottish Schoolsport Federation 26
Scottish Teachers for a New Era 55
self-start skills 54

self-study demands 69
Sharp, B. 8, 11, 13
Sharp, R. 11
Shulman, L. S. 60
Sicilia-Camacho, A. 35
Siedentop, D. 4, 21–2, 43, 59
situated learning 4, 41, 55
skateboarding 32, 65
skills transfer 4, 37
skills-focused teaching 37, 41
Smith, L. B. 58
social inclusion 18
social justice 49
social skills 44
SOED/HMIE 11, 16
specialist teachers, lack of 16
sport 3, 5, 16, 20–1, 22, 52
sport academies 22
Sport Education 4, 45–6, 59, 67
Sport Scotland 24, 25, 27, 63, 66, 72
sports lobby 63–4
sports-based participation 24
sports-related degree programmes 50–1
SQA (Scottish Qualifications Authority) 2, 13, 27, 61
SSCP (School Sport Coordinator Programme) 24, 25, 62, 64, 65
Standage, M. 4
Standard Grades: and CfE 15, 69; gender differences 12; perceptual-motor skills 11; performance/knowledge 8–9; physical activity 10; physical education 68, 71
standards-based approach 56
Stirling University 50
Strathclyde University 50
Stratton, S. 19
Stroot, S. A. 38
student teachers 5, 39, 52, 54, 55
Sutherland Report 58
swimming 42–3
swimming pools 72

tactical approach 4, 44, 67
teacher educators 55
teacher mentors 55
teacher-centred styles 4, 35, 37, 41
teachers: autonomy 56, 59; conditions of service 63; experienced 56–61; as facilitators 43–4, 45; out of school roles 62, 63; seconded 10; support for 73–4; theory 39–40; *see also* physical education teachers
Teaching and Learning Research

Programme 73
Teaching Games for Understanding: *see* TGfU
teaching styles 35, 36, 37–8, 46
team games: categories 44; in curriculum 16, 19, 23, 26; motor skills 36, 41, 44–6; recreational activities 66
team learning 44
technique development 37, 74
TGfU (Teaching Games for Understanding) 4, 44–5, 45–6, 59, 67, 74
Thelen, E. 58
Theodoulides, A. 32
Thomson, I. 8, 10, 11
Thorburn, M. 12, 13, 14, 25, 27, 29, 36, 37, 40, 46, 60, 62, 64, 65, 66, 69, 72
Thorpe, R. 4, 44, 45, 74
3--18 curriculum 17, 29, 58
Treasure, D. 36
Tsangaridou, N. 39, 59
Turner, A. P. 45

Van Driel, J. H. 60
volunteerism 62–3, 75

Wallhead, T. L. 27
Wallian, N. 43
Watt, M. 20–1
Weiss, M. R. 33, 35
Welk, G. J. 33, 34
Whitty, G. 25
Wigfield, A. 47
Williams, A. M. 37
Winning Scotland Foundation 27
Wright, S. 55

Xiang, P. 33

Yelling, M. 59, 60
youth culture 75
youth sport 24–8, 49, 64–7